John Fiske

Tobacco and Alcohol

John Fiske

Tobacco and Alcohol

ISBN/EAN: 9783744662635

Printed in Europe, USA, Canada, Australia, Japan

Cover: Foto ©Andreas Hilbeck / pixelio.de

More available books at **www.hansebooks.com**

TOBACCO AND ALCOHOL

I. IT DOES PAY TO SMOKE.
II. THE COMING MAN WILL DRINK WINE.

BY

JOHN FISKE, M. A., LL. B.

—" *Quæres a me lector amabilis quod plerique sciscitantur laudemne
an vero damnem tabaci usum ? Respondeo tabacum optimum esse. Tu
mi lector tabaco utere non abutere.*"—MAGNENUS Exercitationes de Tabaco, *Ticino,* 1658.

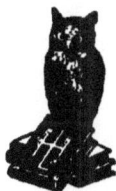

NEW YORK:
LEYPOLDT & HOLT.
1869.

Stereotyped by Little, Rennie & Co.,
430 Broome St., New York.

PREFACE.

Five weeks ago to-day the idea of writing an essay upon the physiological effects of Tobacco and Alcohol had never occurred to us. Nevertheless, the study of physiology and pathology—especially as relating to the action of narcotic-stimulants upon nutrition—has for several years afforded us, from time to time, agreeable recreation. And being called upon, in the discharge of a regularly-recurring duty, to review Mr. Parton's book entitled "Smoking and Drinking," it seemed worth while, in justice to the subject, to go on writing,—until the present volume was the result.

This essay is therefore to be regarded as a review article, rewritten and separately published. It is nothing more, as regards either the time and thought directly bestowed·upon it, or the completeness with which it treats the subject. Bearing this in mind, the reader will understand the somewhat fantastic sub-titles of the book, and the presence of a number of citations and comments which would ordinarily be neither essential nor desirable in a serious discussion. Had we been writing a systematic treatise, with the object of stating exhaustively our theory of the action of Tobacco and Alcohol, we should

have found it needful to be far more abstruse and
technical; and we should certainly have had no occasion whatever to mention Mr. Parton's name.   As
it is, the ideal requirements of a complete statement
have been subordinated—though by no means sacri
ficed—to the obvious desideratum of making a summary at once generally intelligible and briefly conclusive.

The materials used especially in the preparation
of this volume were the following:

Anstie: Stimulants and Narcotics.   Philadelphia, 1865.

Lallemand, Duroy, et Perrin: Du Rôle de l'Alcool et des
Anesthésiques.   Paris, 1860.

Baudot: De la Destruction de l'Alcool dans l'Organisme.
Union Médicale, Nov. et Déc., 1863.

Bouchardat et Sandras: De la Digestion des Boissons Al
cooliques.   Annales de Chimie et de Physique, 1847, tom. xxi.

Duchek: Ueber das Verhalten des Alkohols im thierischen
Organismus.   Vierteljahrschrift für die praktische Heilkunde.
Prague, 1833.

Von Bibra: Die Narkotischen Genussmittel und der Mensch.
Nürnberg, 1855.

And the works of Taylor, Orfila, Christison, and Pereira,
on Materia Medica and Poisons; of Flint, Dalton, Dunglison,
Draper, Carpenter, Liebig, Lehmann, and Moleschott, on
general Physiology; several of the special works on Tobacco mentioned in the Appendix; and the current medical
journals.

Oxford Street, Cambridge, *November* 23, 1868.

TOBACCO AND ALCOHOL.

I.

IT DOES PAY TO SMOKE.

MR. JAMES PARTON having abandoned the habit of smoking, has lately entered upon the task of persuading the rest of mankind to abandon it also.[1] His "victory over himself"—to use the favourite expression—would be incomplete unless followed up by a victory over others; and he therefore desists for a season from his congenial labours in panegyrizing Aaron Burr, B. F. Butler, and other popular heroes, in order that he may briefly descant upon the evil characters of

---

[1] Smoking and Drinking. By James Parton. Boston, Ticknor & Fields, 1868. 12mo, pp. 151.

tobacco and its kindred stimulants. Some
of the sophisms and exaggerations which he
has brought into play while doing so, invite
attention before we attempt what he did not
attempt at all—to state squarely and honest-
ly the latest conclusions of science on the
subject.

According to Mr. Parton, tobacco is responsible for nearly all the ills which in modern times have afflicted humanity. As will
be seen, he makes no half-way work of the
matter. He must have the whole loaf, or he
will not touch a crumb. He scorns all care-
fully-limited, compromising, philosophical statements of the case. Whatever the verdict of
science may turn out to be, he *knows* that
no good ever did come, ever does come, or
ever will come, from the use of tobacco.
All bad things which tobacco can do, as well
as all bad things which it cannot do—all
probable, possible, improbable, impossible, in-
conceivable, and nonsensical evil results—are

by Mr. Parton indiscriminately lumped together and laid at its door. It is simply a
diabolical poison which, since he has happily
eschewed the use of it, had better be at once
extirpated from the face of the earth. Of all
this, Mr. Parton is so very sure that he
evidently thinks any reasoning on the subject
quite superfluous and out of place.

The paucity of his arguments is, however,
compensated by the multitude and hardihood
of his assertions.   A sailor, he says, should
not smoke; for " why should he go round this
beautiful world drugged ?"   Note the *petitio
principii* in the use of the word " drugged."
That the smoker is, in the bad sense of the
word, drugging himself, is the very point to
be determined; but Mr. Parton feels so sure
that he substitutes a sly question - begging
participle for a conscientious course of investigation. With nine readers out of ten this
takes just as well; and then it is so much
easier and safer, you know.   Neither should

soldiers smoke, for the glare of their pipes
may enable some hostile picket to take deadly
aim at them. Moreover, a "forward car," in
which a crowd of smoking veterans are re-
turning from the seat of war, is a disgusting
place. And "that two and two make four is
not a truth more unquestionably certain than
that smoking does diminish a soldier's power
of endurance, and does make him more susceptible to imaginary dangers." (p. 17.) This
statement, by the way, is an excellent specimen of Mr. Parton's favourite style of assertion.
He does not say that his private opinion on
this complex question in nervous physiology
is well supported by observation, experiment
and deduction. He does not say that there
is at least a preponderance of evidence in its
favour. He does not call it as probable as
any opinion on such an intricate matter can
ever be. But he says "it is as unquestionably certain as that two and two make four."
Nothing less will satisfy him. Let it no longer.

be said that, in the difficult science of physiology, absolute certainty is not attainable!

Then again, the soldier should not smoke, because he ought always to be in training; and no Harvard oarsman needs to be told "that smoking reduces the tone of the system and diminishes all the forces of the body—he *knows* it." The profound physiological knowledge of the average Harvard under-graduate it would perhaps seem ungracious to question; but upon this point, be it said with due reverence, doctors disagree. We have known athletes who told a different story. Waiving argument for the present, however, we go on presenting Mr. Parton's "certainties." One of these is that every man should be kept all his life in what prizefighters call "condition," which term Mr. Parton supposes to mean "the natural state of the body, uncontaminated by poison, and unimpaired by indolence or excess." Awhile ago we had "drugs," now we have "poison," but not a

syllable of argument to show that either term
is. properly applicable to tobacco.   But Mr.
Parton's romantic idea of the state of the
body which accompanies training is one which
is likely to amuse, if it does not edify, the
physiologist. So far from "condition" being
the "natural (i. e. healthy) state of the body,"
it is an extremely unnatural state.   It is a
condition which generally exhausts a man by
the time he is thirty-five years old, rendering
him what prizefighters call "stale."   It is not
"natural," or normal, for the powers either of
the muscular or of the nervous system to be
kept constantly at the maximum.   What our
minds and bodies need is intermittent, rhyth-
mical activity.   " In books and work and
healthful play," not "in work and work and
work alway," should our earlier and later years
be passed ; and a man who is always training
for a boatrace is no more likely to hold out in
the plenitude of his powers than a man who
is always studying sixteen hours a day.   The

only reason why our boys at Yale and Harvard are sometimes permanently benefited by their extravagant athleticism is that they usually leave off before it is too late, and begin to live more normally. For the blood to be continually determined toward the muscles, and for the stomach to be continually digesting none but concentrated food, is a state of things by no means favourable to a normal rate and distribution of nutritive action; and it is upon this normal rate and distribution of nutrition that life, health and strength depend. It is as assisting this process that we shall presently show the temperate use of tobacco to be beneficial. Mr. Parton's idea well illustrates the spirit of that species of "radical" philosophy which holds its own opinions as absolutely and universally, not as relatively and partially, true; which, consequently, is incapable of seeing that one man's meat may be another man's poison, and which is unable to steer safely by Scylla without

turning the helm so far as to pitch head fore-
most into Charybdis. Mr. Parton sees that
athletic exercise is healthful, and he jumps at
once to the conclusion that every man should
always and in all circumstances keep himself
in training.   Such was not the theory of the
ancient Athenians : μηδὲν ἄγαν was their
principle of life,—the principle by virtue of
which they made themselves competent to
instruct mankind.

Having thus said his say about muscular
men, Mr. Parton goes on to declare that smoking is a barbarism.   "There is something in the
practice that allies a man with barbarians, and
constantly tends to make him think and talk
like a barbarian."   We suppose Mr. Parton
must *know* this; for he does not attempt to
prove it, unless indeed he considers a rather
stupid anecdote to be proof.   He tells us how
he listened for an hour or so to half a dozen
Yale students in one of the public rooms of a
New-Haven hotel, talking with a stable-keeper

about boat-racing. They swore horribly; and of course Mr. Parton believes that if they had not been smokers they would neither have used profane language nor have condescended to talk with stable-keepers. *Sancta simplicitas!*

" We must admit, too, I think, that smoking dulls a man's sense of the rights of others. Horace Greeley is accustomed to sum up his opinions upon this branch of the subject by saying: 'When a man begins to smoke, he immediately becomes a hog.'" Our keen enjoyment of Mr. Greeley's lightness of touch and refined delicacy of expression should not be allowed to blind us to the possible incompleteness of his generalization. What! Milton a hog? Locke, Addison, Scott, Thackeray, Robert Hall, Christopher North—hogs?

And then smoking is an expensive habit. If a man smoke ten cigars daily, at twenty cents each, his smoking will cost him from seven to eight hundred dollars a year.

This dark view of the case needs to be enlivened by a little contrast. "While at Cambridge the other day, looking about among the ancient barracks in which the students live, I had the curiosity to ask concerning the salaries of the professors in Harvard College." Probably he inquired of a *Goody*, or of one of the *Pocos* who are to be found earning bread by the sweat of their brows in the neighbourhood of these venerable shanties, for it seems they told him that the professors were paid fifteen or eighteen hundred dollars a year. Had he taken the trouble to step into the steward's office, he might have learned that they are paid three thousand dollars a year. Such is the truly artistic way in which Mr. Parton makes contrasts—$1500 *per annum* for a professor, $800 for cigars! Therefore, it does not pay to smoke.

Smoking, moreover, makes men slaves. The Turks and Persians are great smokers, and they live under a despotic form of government. Q. E. D. The extreme liberality of Oriental institutions *before* the introduction of tobacco Mr. Parton probably thinks so well known as not to require mention. But still worse, the Turks and Persians are great despisers of women; and this is evidently because they smoke. For woman and tobacco are natural enemies. The most perfect of men, the "highly-groomed" Goethe—as Mr. Parton elegantly calls him—loved women and hated tobacco. This aspect of the question is really a serious one. Tobacco, says our reformer, is woman's rival,—and her successful rival; therefore she hates it. For as Mr. Parton, with profound insight into the mysteries of the feminine character, gravely observes, "women do not disapprove their rivals; they hate them." This "ridiculous brown leaf," then, is not only in general the cause of all evil, but in particular it is the foe of woman. "It takes off the edge of virility "!!² It makes us regard woman from the Black Crook point of view. If it had not been for tobacco, that wretched phantasmagoria would not have had a run of a dozen nights. " Science" justifies this conjecture, and even if it did not, Mr. Parton intimates that he should make it. Doubtless!

One bit of Mr. Parton's philosophy still

---

² When we first read this remark, we took it for a mere burst of impassioned rhetoric; but on second thoughts, it appears to have a meaning. Another knight-errant in physiology charges tobacco with producing " giddiness, sickness, vomiting, vitiated taste of the mouth, loose bowels, diseased liver, congestion of the brain, apoplexy, palsy, mania, loss of memory, amaurosis, deafness, nervousness, *emasculation*, and cowardice." Lizars, *On Tobacco*, p. 29. A goodly array of bugbears, quite aptly illustrating the remark of one of our medical professors, that hygienic reformers, in the length of their lists of imaginary diseases, are excelled only by the itinerant charlatans who vend panaceas. There is, however, no scientific foundation for the statement that tobacco " takes off the edge of virility." The reader who is interested in this question may consult Orfila, *Toxicologie*, tom. II. p. 527; *Annales d'Hygiène*, tom. XXXVIII.; and a Memoir by Laycock in the *London Medical Gazette*, 1846, tom. III.

calls for brief comment. He wishes to speak of the general tendency of the poor man's pipe; and he means to say " that it tends to make him satisfied with a lot which it is his chief and immediate duty to alleviate,—he ought to hate and loathe his tenement-house home." A fine specimen of the dyspeptic philosophy of radicalism! Despise all you have got, because you cannot have something better. We believe it is sometimes described as the philosophy of progress. There can of course be no doubt that Mr. Parton's hod-carrier will work all the better next day, if he only spends the night in fretting and getting peevish over his "tenement-house home."

Such then, in sum and substance, is our reformer's indictment against tobacco. It lowers the tone of our systems, and it makes us contented; it wastes money, it allies us with barbarians, and it transforms us—*mira quadam metamorphosi*—into swine. Goethe, therefore, did not smoke, the Coming Man will not smoke, and General Grant, with tardy repentance, " has reduced his daily allowance of cigars." And as for Mr. Buckle, the author of an able book which Mr. Parton rather too enthusiastically calls " the most valuable work of this century,"—if Mr. Buckle had but lived, he would doubtless have inserted a chapter in his "History," in which tobacco would have been ranked with theology, as one of the obstacles to civilization.

Throughout Mr. Parton's rhapsody, the main question, the question chiefly interesting to every one who smokes or wishes to smoke, is uniformly slurred over. Upon the question whether it is unhealthy to smoke, the Encyclopædias which Mr. Parton has consulted do not appear to have helped him to an answer. Yet this is a point which, in making up our minds about the profitableness of smoking, must not be taken for granted, but scientifically tested.

What, then, does physiology say about this notion — rather widespread in countries over which Puritanism has passed—that the use of tobacco is necessarily or usually injurious to health? Simply that it is a popular delusion—a delusion which even a moderate acquaintance with the first principles of modern physiology cannot fail to dissipate. Nay, more; if our interpretation shall prove to be correct, it goes still further. It says that smoking, so far from being detrimental to health, is, in the great majority of cases, where excess is avoided, beneficial to health; in short, that the careful and temperate smoker is, other things equal, likely to be more vigorous, more cheerful, and more capable of prolonged effort than the man who never smokes.

We do not pretend to *know* all this, nor are we "as certain of it as that two and two make four." Such certainty, though desirable, is not to be had in complex physiological questions. But we set down these propositions as being,

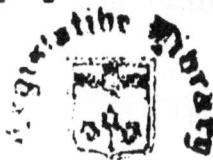

so far as we can make out, in the present
state of science, the verdict of physiology in
the matter. Future inquiry may reverse that
verdict; but as the physiologic evidence now
stands, there is a quite appreciable preponderance in favor of the practice of smoking. Such
was our own conclusion long before we had
ever known, or cared to know, the taste of a
cigar or pipe; and such it remains after eight
years' experience in smoking. We shall en-
deavor concisely to present the *rationale* of the
matter, dealing with some general doctrines
likely to assist us both now and later, when we
come to speak of alcohol.

We do not suppose it necessary to overhaul
and quote all that the illustrious Pereira, in his
"Materia Medica,"[3] and Messrs. Johnston and

---

[3] "I am not acquainted with any well-ascertained ill effects resulting from the habitual practice of smoking."—
Pereira, *Materia Medica*, vol. ii., p. 1431. Tobacco "is
used in immense quantities over the whole world as an article of luxury, without any bad effect having ever been
clearly traced to it."—Christison on *Poisons*, p. 730. These

Lewes, in their deservedly popular books, have said about the physiologic action of tobacco. Their works may easily be consulted by any one who is interested in the subject; and their verdict is in the main confined to the general proposition that, from the temperate use of tobacco in smoking, no deleterious results have ever been proved to follow. More modern and far more elaborate data for forming an opinion are to be found in the great treatise of Dr. Anstie, on " Stimulants and Narcotics," which we shall make the basis of the following argument.[4]

In the first place, we want some precise definition of the quite vaguely understood word,

---

two short sentences, from such consummate masters of their science as Christison and Pereira, should far more than outweigh all the volumes of ignorant denunciation which have been written by crammers, smatterers, and puritanical reformers, from King James down.

[4] Only a basis, however. The argument as applied to tobacco, though a necessary corollary from Dr. Anstie's doctrines, is in no sense Dr. Anstie's argument. We are ourselves solely responsible for it.

"narcotic." What is a narcotic? *A narcotic is any poison which, when taken in sufficient quantities into the system, produces death by paralysis.* The tyro in physiology knows that death must start either from the lungs, the heart, or the nervous system. Now a narcotic is anything which, in due quantity, kills by killing the nervous system. When death is caused by too great a proportion of carbonic acid in the air, it begins at the lungs; but when it is caused by a dose of prussic acid, it begins at the medulla oblongata, the death of which causes the heart and lungs to stop acting. Prussic acid is, therefore, a narcotic; and so are strychnine, belladonna, aconite, nicotine, sulphuric ether, chloroform, alcohol, opium, thorn-apple, betel, hop, lettuce, tea, coffee, coca, hemp, chocolate, and many other substances. All these, taken in requisite doses, will kill by paralysis; and all of them, taken in lesser but considerable doses, will induce a state of the nerves known as narcosis, which is

nothing more nor less than incipient paralysis.
Every man who smokes tobacco, or drinks tea
or coffee, until his hands are tremulous and his
stomach-nerves slightly depressed, has just
started on the road to paralysis : he may never
travel farther on it, but he has at least turned
the corner. Every man who drinks ale, wine,
or spirit until his face is flushed and his forehead moist, has slightly paralyzed himself.
Alcoholic drunkenness is paralysis. The mental and emotional excitement, falsely called
exaltation, is due, not to stimulation, but to
paralysis of the cerebrum. The unsteady gait
and groping motion of the hands are due to
paralysis of the cerebellum. The feverish pulse
and irregular respiration are due to paralysis
of the medulla oblongata. The flushed face
and tremulous, distressed stomach, are due to
paralysis of the sympathetic ganglia. And
when a person is "dead-drunk," his inability
to perform the ordinary reflex acts of locomo-
tion and grasping is due in part to paralysis

of the spinal centres. The coma, or so-called sleep of drunkenness, is perfectly distinct from true reparative sleep, being the result of serious paralysis of the cerebrum, and closely allied to delirium.[5] Now, what we have stated in detail concerning alcohol is also true of tobacco. A fatal dose of nicotine kills, just like prussic acid, by paralyzing the medulla, and thus stopping the heart's beating. The

---

[5] Sleep is caused by a diminution of blood in the cerebrum; stupor and delirium, as well as *insomnia*, or nocturnal wakefulness, are probably caused by excess of blood in the cerebrum. We feel sleepy after a heavy meal, because the stomach, intestines and liver appropriate blood which would ordinarily be sent to the brain. But after a drunken debauch, a man sinks in stupor because the brain is partially congested. The blood rushes to the paralyzed part, just as it rushes to an inflamed part; and in the paralysis, as in the inflammation, nutrition and the products of nutrition are lowered. The habitual drunkard lowers the quality of his nervous system, and impairs its sensitiveness,—hence the necessity of increasing the dose. It will be seen, therefore, that it is not the function of a narcotic, as such, to induce sleep, though in a vast number of cases it may induce stupor. The headache felt on awaking from stupor, is the index of impaired nutrition, quite the reverse of the vigor felt on arising from sleep.

ordinary narcotic dose does not produce such notable effects as the dose of alcohol, because it is hardly possible to take enough of it. Excessive smoking does not make a man maudlin, but it causes restless wakefulness, which is a symptom of cerebral paralysis, and is liable, in rare cases, to end in coma. Its action on the cerebellum and spinal cord cannot be readily stated; but its effect on the medulla and sympathetic is most notable, being seen in depression or feeble acceleration of the pulse, trembling, nausea of the stomach, and torpidity of the liver and intestines. Nearly or quite all of these effects producible by tobacco, are producible also, in even a heightened degree, by narcotic doses of tea and coffee. A concentrated dose of tea will produce a paralytic shock; and a single cup of very strong coffee is sometimes enough to cause alarming disorder in the heart's action. All these narcotic effects, we repeat, are instances of paralytic depression. *In no case*

*are they instances of stimulus followed by re-
action ; but whenever a narcotic dose is taken,
the depressive paralytic action begins as soon as
the dose is absorbed by the blood-vessels.* The
cheerful and maudlin drunkard is not under
the action of stimulus. His rapid, irregular,
excited mental action is no more entitled to
be called "exaltation" than is the delirium
of typhoid fever. In the one case and in
the other, we have not stimulation but depression of the vitality of the cerebrum ; in
both cases, the nutrition is seriously impaired ;
in both cases, molecular disorganization of the
nerve-material is predominant.

So much concerning narcotics has been established, with vast and profound learning, by
Dr. Anstie. No doubt, by this time, the reader
is beginning to rub his eyes and ask, Is this
the way in which you are going to show that
smoking is beneficial? You define tobacco as
a poison which causes paralysis, and then as-
sure us that it pays to smoke! It is true,

this has at first sight a paradoxical look; but
as the reader proceeds further, he will see that
we are not indulging either in paradoxes or
in sophisms. We wish him to take nothing
for granted, but merely to follow attentively
our exposition of the case. We have indeed
called tobacco a poison,—and so it is, if taken
in narcotic doses. We have accused it of producing paralysis,—and so it does, when taken
in adequate narcotic doses. We would now
call attention to a property of narcotics, which
is well enough known to all physiologists, but
is usually quite misapprehended or ignored by
popular writers on alcohol and tobacco.[6] We

---

[6] Mr. Lizars (*On Tobacco*, p. 54) has the impudence
to cite Pereira (vol. ii. p. 1426) as an opponent of
smoking, because he calls nicotine a deadly poison!
And on p. 58 he similarly misrepresents Johnston.
This is the way in which popular writers contrive to
marshal an array of scientific authorities on their side.
In the case of tobacco, however, it is difficult to find
physiologists who will justify the popular clamour. They
have a way of taking the opposite view; and when
Mr. Lizars cannot get rid of them in any other way,
he insinuates that all writings in favour of tobacco

allude to the fact that narcotics, when taken in certain small quantities, do not behave as narcotics, but as *stimulants;* and that they will in such cases produce the exact reverse of a narcotic effect. Instead of lowering nutrition, they will raise it; instead of paralyzing, they will invigorate. Taken in a stimulant dose, tobacco is not only not a producer, it is an averter, of paralysis. It is not only not a poison, but it is a healthful, reparatory stimulus.

It is desirable that this point should be thoroughly understood before wè advance a step farther. Here is the *pons asinorum* in the study of narcotics, but it must be crossed if we would get at the truth concerning alcohol and

---

"have been *got up* from more than questionable motives." (p. 137.) This is in the richest vein of what, for want of a better word, we have called radicalism; and may be compared with Mr. Parton's belief that physicians recommend alcoholic drinks because they like to fatten on human suffering! (*Smoking and Drinking*, p. 56.)

tobacco. Alcohol is a poison, says the teetotaler, who means well, but has not studied the human organism ; alcohol is a poison, and once a poison always a poison. Nothing can seem more logical or reasonable, so long as one knows nothing about the subject. A quart of brandy is admitted to be poison; is not, therefore, a spoonful of brandy also poison? We reply, by no means. Physiological questions are not to be settled by formal logic. Here the quantity is the all-essential element to be taken into the account. Common salt, in large doses, is a virulent poison ; in lesser doses it is a powerful emetic; in small doses it is a gentle stimulant, and an article of food absolutely essential to the maintenance of life. In the spirit of the teetotaler's logic, then, it may be asked, If a pound of salt is a poison, is not a grain of salt also a poison? We reply, call it what you please, you cannot support life without it. So from the poisonous character of the quart of brandy, the poisonous character of the spoonful is by no means a legitimate inference. The evil effects of the small dose are to be ascertained by experiment, not to be taken for granted. Logic is useful in the hands of those who understand the subject they reason about; but in other hands it sometimes leads to queer results. It was logic that used up the one-hoss shay.

The general principle to guide us here is that of Claude Bernard, that whatever substance or action, in due amount, tends to improve nutrition, may, in excessive amount, tend to damage nutrition. In the vast majority of cases the difference between food and poison, between beneficent and malignant action, is only a difference of quantity. Oxygen is the all-important stimulus, without which nutrition could not be carried on for a moment. It constitutes about one-fifth of our atmospheric air. Let us now step into an atmosphere of pure oxygen, and we shall speedily rue such a radical proceeding. We shall live so fast that waste will soon get ahead of repair, and our strength will be utterly exhausted. The effect of sunlight on the optic nerve is to stimulate the medulla, and increase thereby the vigor of the circulation. But too intense a glare produces blindness and dizziness. The carpenter's thumb, by friction against the tools he uses, becomes over-nourished and tough; but if the friction be too continuous, there is lowered nutrition and inflammation. Moderate exercise enlarges the muscles; exercise carried beyond the point of fatigue wastes them. The stale prize-fighter and the overworked farmer are, from a physical point of view, pitiable specimens of manhood. A due amount of rich food strengthens the system and renders it superior to disease; an excessive amount of rich food weakens the system, and opens the door for all manner of aches and ailments. A pinch of mustard, eaten with meat, stimulates the lining of the stomach, and probably aids digestion; but a mustard poultice lowers the vitality of

any part to which it is applied. Moderate
emotional excitement is a healthful stimulus,
both to mind and body; but intense and prolonged excitement is liable to produce delirium, mania, or paralysis. *Ne quid nimis,*
therefore, the maxim of the wise epicurean,
is also the golden rule of hygiene. If you
would keep a sound mind in a sound body,
do not rush to extremes. Steer cautiously
between Scylla and Charybdis, and do not get
wrecked upon the one or swallowed up in the
other.

Few persons who have not been specially
educated in science have ever learned this
great lesson of Materia Medica, "that everything depends on the size of the dose." It
is not merely that a small dose will often
produce effects differing in degree from those
produced by a large dose; nor is it merely
that the small dose will often produce an effect differing in kind from that of the large
dose; but it is that the small dose will often

produce effects diametrically opposite and antagonistic to those of the large dose. The small dose may even serve as a partial antidote to the large dose. The adage concerning the hair of the dog that has bitten us, embodies the empirical wisdom of our ancestors on this subject. Especially is this true of all the substances classed as narcotics. In doses of a certain size, they, one and all, produce effects exactly the reverse of narcotic. If anything is entitled to be called a deadly narcotic poison, it is strychnia, which, by paralyzing the spinal cord, induces tetanic convulsions: yet minute doses of strychnia have been used with signal success in the cure of hemiplegic paralysis. In teething children, the pressure upon the dental branches of the trigeminal nerve sometimes causes an irritation so great as partly to paralyze the medulla, inducing clonic convulsions, and perhaps death by interference

with the heart's action.[7] In these cases,
alcohol has been frequently used with notable efficacy, averting as it does the paralysis
of the medulla. Epileptic fits, choreic convulsions, and muscular spasms—such as colic,
and spasmodic asthma—are also often re-
lieved by the tonic or anti-paralytic action
of alcohol. And how often has the temperate
smoker, after some occasion of distressing
excitement, his limbs and viscera trembling,
his nerves " all unstrung," or incipiently paralyzed,—how often has the temperate smoker
found his whole system soothed and quieted,
and the steadiness of his nerves restored, by
a single pipe of tobacco! That this is due
to its action as a counteracter of paralysis is
shown by the fact that tobacco has been
successfully used in tetanus,[8] in spasm of

---

[7] Clendon, *On the Causes of the Evils of Infant Den-
tition.*

[8] Curling, *On Tetanus*, p. 168; Earle, in *Med. Chir.
Trans.*, vol. vi., p. 92; and O'Beirne, in *Dublin Hospital
Reports.* vols. i. and ii.

rima glottidis,[9] in spasmodic asthma,[10] and in epilepsy.[11] For these phænomena physiology has but one explanation. They are due to the fact that narcotics, in small doses, either nourish, or facilitate the normal nutrition of the nervous system. They restore its equilibrium, enabling it, with diminished effort, to discharge its natural functions. And anything which performs this office is, in modern physiology, called a *stimulant.*

Here then we have obtained an important amendment of our notion of a narcotic. A narcotic is a substance which, taken in the requisite dose, causes paralysis. But we have seen that by diminishing the dose we at last reach a point where the narcotic entirely ceases to act as a narcotic and becomes a stimulant. What then is a stimulant? There is a prejudice afloat which interferes

---

[9] Wood, *U. S. Dispensatory.*
[10] Sigmond, in *Lancet,* vol. ii., p. 253.
[11] Currie, *Med. Rep.,* vol. i., p. 163.

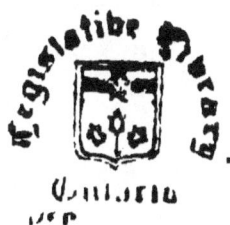

with the proper apprehension of this word.
People call alcohol, indiscriminately, a stimulant; and when a man gets drunk, he is
incorrectly said to be stimulating himself
stimulants are therefore looked at askance,
as things which demoralize. The reader is
already in a position to know better than this.
He sees already that it is not stimulus but
narcosis which is ruining the drunkard.
Nevertheless, that he may understand thoroughly what a stimulant is, we must give
further explanation and illustration.

Food and stimulus are the two great,
equally essential factors or co-efficients in the
process of nutrition. We mean by this, that
in order to nourish your system and make
good its daily waste, you need both food
and stimulus. You must have both, or you
cannot support life. Day by day, in every
act of life, be it in the acts of working and
thinking which go on consciously, or be it in
the acts of digestion and respiration which

go on unconsciously, in the mere keeping ourselves alive, we are continually using up and rendering worthless the materials of which our bodies are composed. We use up tissue as an engine uses up fuel; and we therefore need constant coaling. Tissue once used is no better than ashes; it must be excreted, and food must be taken to form new tissue. Now the wonderful process by which digested food is taken up from the blood by the tissues—each tissue taking just what will serve it and no more, muscle-making stuff to muscle, bone-making stuff to bone, nerve-making stuff to nerve—is called assimilation, nutrition, or repair. It is according as waste or repair predominates that we are feeble or strong, useless or efficient. When repair is greatly in excess, as it usually is in childhood and youth, we grow. When waste is greatly in excess, we die of consumption, gangrene, or starvation. When the daily repair slightly outweighs the daily waste, we are healthy and vigorous. When the daily repair is not quite enough to replace the daily waste, we are feeble, easily wearied, and liable to be assailed by some illness.

Now, in order to carry on this great process of nutrition, we have said that food and stimulus are equally indispensable. We must have food or we can have nothing to assimilate ; but we must also have stimulus, or no assimilation will take place. *The unstimulated tissue will not assimilate food.* The nutritive material rushes by it, unsought for and unappropriated, and no repair takes place. There are some people whom no amount of eating will build up : what they need is not more food, but more nerve stimulus; they doubtless eat already more than their tissues are able to assimilate. In pulmonary consumption, the chief monster which we have to fight against is impaired nutrition, the tubercles being only a secondary and derivative symptom.[12] The problem before us, in dealing with consumption, is to improve nutrition, to make the tissues assimilate food. And to this end we prescribe, for example, whisky and milk—a food which easily reaches the tissues, and a stimulant which urges them to take up the food sent to them. We define, therefore, a stimulant as *any substance which, brought to bear in proper quantities upon the nervous system, facilitates nutrition.*

At the head of all stimulants stands oxygen, concerning which, for further illustration, we shall quote the following passage from Dr. Anstie :

"It needs but a glance at the vital condition of different populations in any country to arrive at a tolerably correct idea of the virtues of oxygen as a promoter of health and a curer

---

[12] Indeed, there are many fatal cases in which tubercles never appear. See Niemeyer on *Pulmonary Phthisis.*

of disease. If we compare the physical condition of the inhabitants of a London alley,
an agricultural village, and a breezy sea-side
hamlet, we shall recognize the truth of the
description which assigns to it the same ther-
apeutic action as is exercised by drugs, to
which the name of stimulant seems more nat-
urally applicable than to such a familiar agent
as one which we are constantly breathing in
the common air. A child that has been bred
in a London cellar may be taken to possess
a constitution which is a type of all the evil
tendencies which our stimulants are intended
to obviate. . . . . It is highly suggestive
to find that that very same quiet and perfect
action of the vital functions, without undue
waste, without pain, and without *excessive* material growth, is precisely what we produce,
when we produce any useful effect, by the
administration of stimulants, though, as
might be expected, our artificial means are
weak and uncertain in their operation,

compared with the great natural stimulus of life."[13]

Stimulus implies no undue exaltation of the activity of any part of the organism. In complete health all parts of the body should work together in unhindered co-operation. Any undue exaltation of a particular function—excessive brain-action, excessive muscular-nutrition, excessive deposit of fat—is a symptom of lowered life, in which the co-ordinating control of the whole system over its several parts is diminished. Stimulus, on the other hand, implies an increase of the co-ordinating and controlling power. Dr. Anstie therefore recommends that the word "overstimulation" be disused, as unphilosophical and self-contradictory.

In yet one further particular, current notions need to be rectified before we can proceed. *In no case is the action of a stimulant followed by a depressive reaction.* This

---

[13] *Stimulants and Narcotics*, p. 144.

seems at first like a paradox. Physiologists
have in times past maintained the contrary;
and some have even ventured to apply to the
phænomena of stimulation the dynamic law
that "action and reaction are equal and opposite." But in physiology we shall not be
helped much by the theorems of mechanics.
In no case is the stimulus followed by any
other "recoil" than that which is implied in
the mere gradual cessation of its action, just
as in the case of food which has been eaten,
assimilated, and used up. We quote the following from Dr. Anstie :—"We often hear the
effects of strong irritation of the skin, or the
mucous surfaces, quoted as an example of the
way in which action and reaction follow each
other. The immediate effect of such treat-
ment (it is said) is to quicken the circulation
and improve the vital condition of the part,
but its *ultimate* result is a complete stagnation
of the vital activities in the irritated tissues.
The real explanation of the matter is, however,

very different. Mild stimulation of the skin
(as by friction, warm liniments, &c.) has no
tendency to produce subsequent depression ;
nor has mild stimulation of the mucous membranes (as by the mustard we eat with our
roast beef). But the application of an irritant
strong enough to produce a morbid depression
at all, produces it *from the first.* Thus the can-
tharidine of a blister has no sooner become
absorbed through the epidermis than it *at
once* deprives a certain area of tissue of its
vitality to a considerable extent, as is explained by the researches of Mr. Lister. . . .
Here is no stimulation first and depressive
recoil afterward, but unmitigated depression
from the first." " What has been commonly
spoken of as the *recoil* from the stimulant
action of a true narcotic is, in fact, simply
the advent of narcosis owing to a large im-
pregnation of the blood with the agent after

---

[14] *Stimulants and Narcotics*, p. 148.

the occurrence of stimulation, owing to a small one. Thus a man drinking four ounces or six ounces of brandy gradually, has not in reality taken a truly narcotic dose till perhaps half the evening has worn away; previously to that he has not been 'indulging in narcotism' at all; nor, had he stopped then, would any after depression have followed, for he might have taken no more than two ounces of brandy, equal perhaps to one ounce of alcohol. But he chose to swallow the extra two ounces or four ounces, thus impregnating his blood with a narcotic mixture capable of acting upon nervous tissue so as to render it incapable of performing its proper functions. *The narcosis has no relation to the stimulation but one of accidental sequence. This is proved by the fact that in cases where a narcotic dose is absorbed with great rapidity, no signs of preliminary stimulation occur."* [15]

---

[15] Id. p. 224.

This disposes of the popular objection to stimulants—based upon the long - exploded theories of vitalistic physiology[16]—that every stimulus is followed by a reaction. It is seen that when a man feels ill and depressed after the use of alcohol or tobacco, it is because he has not stimulated but narcotized himself. We challenge any person, not hopelessly dyspeptic, to produce from his own experience any genuine instance of physical or mental depression as the result of a half-pint of pure

---

[16] "The origin of the belief that stimulation is necessarily followed by a depressive recoil is obviously to be found in the old vitalistic ideas. It is our old acquaintance, the Archæus, whose exhaustion, after his violent efforts in resentment of the goadings which he has endured, is represented in modern phraseology by the term 'depressive reaction.' This idea once being firmly established in the medical mind, the change from professed vitalism to dynamical explanations of physiology has not materially shaken its hold." Id. p. 146. An interesting example of the way in which quite obsolete and forgotten theories will continue clandestinely to influence men's conclusions. The subject is well treated by Lemoine, *Le Vitalisme et l'Animisme de Stahl.* Paris, 1864.

wine taken with his dinner,"[17] or of one or two pipes of mild tobacco smoked after it.

Let us not, however, indulge in sweeping statements. We have expressed ourselves with caution, but a still further limitation needs to be made. There are a few persons who are never stimulated, but always poisonously depressed, by certain particular narcotics. There are a few persons—ourselves among the number—in whom a very temperate dose of coffee will often give rise to well-defined symptoms of narcosis. There are others in whom even the smallest quantity of alcoholic liquor will produce giddiness and flushing of the face. And there are still others upon whom tobacco, no matter how minute the dose, acts as a narcotic poison. But such cases are extremely rare; and it is needless to urge that such persons should conscientiously refrain, once

---

[17] "From good wine, in moderate quantities, there is no reaction whatever."—Brinton, *Treatise on Food and Digestion.*

and always, from the use of the narcotic which thus injuriously affects them. Our friendly challenge, above given, is addressed to the vast majority of people; and thus limited, it may be allowed to stand.

We have now defined a narcotic; we have seen that narcotics, in certain doses, will act as stimulants, and we have defined a stimulant. Until one's ideas upon these points are rendered precise, there is little hope of understanding the ordinary healthy action either of tobacco or of alcohol. But the reader who has followed us thus far will find himself sufficiently prepared for the special inquiry into the stimulant effects of these substances. Confining ourselves, for the present, to tobacco, we shall find that by assisting the nutritive reparatory process, it conforms throughout to the definition of a true stimulant.

What do we do to ourselves when we smoke a cigar or pipe? In the first place, we stimulate, or increase the normal molecular

activity of, the sympathetic system of nerves.
By so doing we slightly increase the secretion
of saliva, and of the gastric,[18] pancreatic, and
intestinal juices.   We accomplish these all-
important secretory actions with a smaller
discharge of nerve force : we economize nerve
force in digestion.   And by this we mean to
say that we perform the work of digesting
food just as well as before, and still have more
of the co-ordinating and controlling nerve-
power left with which to perform the other
functions of life.   Thus at the outset tobacco
exhibits itself as an *economizer of life*.   Such is
the inevitable inference from its stimulant action on the sympathetic.   From the distribution of the sympathetic fibres, we deem it a
fair inference that the bile-secreting function

---

[18] " It is a positive fact that the gastric secretion can
at any time be produced by simply stimulating the salivary glands with tobacco."—Lewes, *Physiology of Common
Life*, vol. i. p. 192.   The gastric secretion is also stimulated
by the action of tobacco on the pneumogastric or eighth
pair of nerves.

of the liver is also facilitated; but of this
there is less direct evidence.[19] We can now
understand why a pipe or cigar dissipates the
feeling of heaviness ensuing upon a dinner, or
other hearty meal; and when we recollect how
instant is the relief, we can form some notion
of the amount of nerve-force which is thus
liberated from the task of digestion. We are
thus also reminded of the hygienic rule that
smoking must be done after eating, and not,
in ordinary cases, upon an empty stomach.
If we smoke when the stomach is empty and
quiescent, the stimulated secretion of the alimentary juices is physiologically wasteful; and,
moreover, the much more rapid absorption of

---

[19] A possible means of testing this inference would be
the judicious employment of smoking as a dietetic
measure in cases of jaundice. This distressing disease
occurs when the torpid liver secretes too little bile. The
biliverdine, which would ordinarily be taken up to make
bile, remains in the blood until, seeking egress through
the sweat-glands, it colours the skin yellow. In the case
of novices, however, great care would need to be taken;
as unskilful smoking is very likely to induce narcosis.

nicotine by the blood-vessels increases the liability to narcotic effects. It is upon this very
principle that the same amount of wine may
stimulate at dinner, but narcotize when taken
in the forenoon.

Thus far we find tobacco to be a friend
and not an enemy. Now, in the second place,
when we smoke, we stimulate the medulla
oblongata, and through this we send a wave
of stimulus down the pneumogastric nerve,
and this makes the heart's action easier. One
of the earliest stimulant effects of tobacco to
be noted is the slightly increased frequency
and strength of the pulse.[20] A narcotic dose
produces quite the opposite effect. It begins
by greatly increasing the frequency while diminishing the strength, so as to make a feeble,
fluttering pulse; and it ends by reducing the
frequency likewise. After some years of tem-

---

[20] See a paper by Dr. E. Smith, read before the British
Association in 1862.

perate smoking we accidentally felt, for the
first time, the narcotic effects of tobacco.
Eight or nine cigars (large twenty-cent ones,
such as Mr. Parton delights in the recollection
of) smoked consecutively while taking a cold
midnight drive, were followed by unmistakable
symptoms of narcosis. Along with the muscular tremour of the stomach, much more acute
than that of ordinary nausea, it was observed
that the pulse, normally strong and regular at
80, had been reduced to 69, and was feeble
and flickering. Similar, no doubt, are the
symptoms which ordinarily worry the novice,
in whom acute narcosis is liable to result from
the lack of skill with which he draws in too
large a quantity of the narcotic constituents
of his cigar. The effects of tobacco, through
the medulla and pneumogastric, upon the
heart, are among its most notable effects. A
dose of pure nicotine stops the heart instantly,
a narcotic dose interferes with its action, but
a stimulant dose facilitates it. The same re-

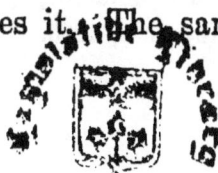

sults are attainable by means of electricity.[21] A powerful current through the pneumogastric of a frog or rabbit will stop the heart, a less powerful current will slacken it, a slight current will somewhat accelerate it. Emotional effects are precisely similar. Sudden overwhelming joy or sorrow may operate as a true narcotic, arresting the heart's contractions, while steady diffusive pleasure always facilitates them.

The stimulant action of tobacco upon the heart is precisely the same as that of sunlight, which, by inciting the nervous expanse of the retina, indirectly strengthens and accelerates the pulse. So far as the circulation is concerned, there is no difference between the two. The one stimulus may indeed be popularly called "natural," while the other is called "artificial," but such a distinction is physiologically meaningless. The

---

[21] See an admirable paper by Lewes in the *Fortnightly Review*, May 15th, 1865.

molecular action is the same and the consequences to the organism are the same in both
cases. The heart's normal action being facilitated, the blood is poured more vigorously
through every artery, every vein, and every
network of capillaries. Every tissue receives
with greater promptness its quota of assimil-
able nutriment. And, the web-like plexuses
of nerve-fibres distributed throughout the
tissues being simultaneously stimulated, the
work of nutrition goes on with enhanced
vigour and efficacy. Nor is it possible for
the excreting organs to escape the influence.
Lungs, skin, and kidneys must be alike in-
cited; and the removal from the blood of
noxious disintegrated matters, the products of
organic waste, is thus hastened.

So much is to be inferred from the stimulant action of tobacco upon the medulla.
Of all this complicated benefit, the brain receives perhaps the largest share. The brain
receives one-fifth, or according to some au-

thorities one-third, of all the blood that is pumped from the heart. More than any other organ it demands for its due nutrition a prompt supply of arterial blood; and more than any other organ it partakes of the advantages resulting from vigorous circulation.

The stimulant action of tobacco upon the spinal cord and the cerebral hemispheres is less conspicuous. Yet even here its familiar influence in stilling nervous tremour and allaying nocturnal wakefulness is good testimony to its essentially beneficent character. Wakefulness and tremour are alike symptoms of diminished vitality; and the agent which removes them is not to be called, as Mr. Parton in his mediæval language calls it, "hostile to the vital principle."

So much for the net results of the stimulant action of tobacco. So far we have travelled on firm ground, and we have not found much to countenance Mr. Parton's view of the subject. But now some curious inquirer may ask, what *is* this stimulant action? What is the physiological expression for it, reduced to its lowest terms? Here we must keep still, or else venture upon ground that is very unfamiliar and somewhat hypothetical. There is no help for it; for we cannot yet give the physiological expression for unstimulated nervous action, reduced to its lowest terms. We know what kind of work nerves perform, but how they perform it we can as yet only guess. Nor, as far as the practical bearings of our subject are concerned, does it matter whether this abstruse point be settled or not. Still, even upon this dark subject recent research has thrown some gleams of light. A nerve-centre is a place where force is liberated by the lapse of the chemically-unstable nerve-molecules into a state of relative stability.[22] To raise

---

[22] We fear that this explanation will be rather unintelligible to the general reader. But it is hardly practicable for us to insert here a disquisition on physiological

them to their previous unstable state, thereby enabling them to fall again and liberate more force, is the function of food. Now our own hypothesis is, that tobacco and other narcotic stimulants enable force to be liberated by the isomeric transformation of the highly complex nerve-molecules, which retain in the process their state of relative instability, and are thus left competent to send forth a second discharge of force without the aid of food.

In support of this hypothesis we have the well-known fact that tobacco, like tea, coffee, alcohol and coca, universally retards organic waste. These substances effect this result in all the tissues, and more especially may they be expected to accomplish it in nervous tissue, where their action is so conspicuously manifest.

---

chemistry. Those who are familiar with modern physiology will readily catch our meaning. Those who are not may skip, if they choose, this parenthetical paragraph.

Thus is explained the familiar action of narcotic-stimulants in relieving weariness. Weariness, in its origin, is either muscular or nervous. It implies a diminution—owing to failing nutrition—of the total amount of contractile or of nervous force in the organism; and it shows that the weary person must either go to sleep or eat something. Now every one knows how a cup of tea, a glass of wine, or a cigar, dispels weariness. Of the three agents, tobacco is perhaps the most efficacious, and it can produce its effect in only one way—namely, by economizing nervous force, and arresting the disintegration of tissue.

Thus also is explained the marvellous food-action of these substances. Tea and coffee enable a man to live on less beefsteak. The Peruvian mountaineer, chewing his coca-leaf, accomplishes incredibly long tramps without stopping to eat. And every hardy soldier, in spite of Mr. Parton, has that within him which tells him that he can better endure

3*

severe marches and wearisome picket-service if he now and then lights his pipe. The personal experience of any one man is, we are aware, not always conclusive; but our own, so far as it goes, bears out the general conclusion. It was when we were engaged in severe daily mental labour, that we first conceived the idea of employing tobacco as a means of husbanding our resources. Narcosis being steadily avoided, the experiment was completely, even unexpectedly, successful. Not only was the daily fatigue sensibly diminished, but the recurrent periods of headache, gloom, and nervous depression were absolutely and finally done away with. That this result was due to improved nutrition was shown by the fact that, during the first three months after the habit of smoking was adopted, the average weight of the body was increased by twenty-four pounds —an increase which has been permanent. No other dietetic or hygienic change was made at the time, by which the direct effects of the tobacco might have been complicated and obscured.

The statement that smoking increases the average weight of the body[23] is not, however, universally true. We have here an excellent illustration of the impracticability of laying down sweeping rules in physiology. Many persons find their weight notably diminished by the use of tobacco; and we frequently hear it said that smoking will not do for thin people, although for those who are fleshy it may not be injurious. In this there is a very natural but very gross confusion of ideas, which a little reflection upon the subject will readily clear up. It is true that moderate smoking sometimes increases

[23] "Tobacco, when the food is sufficient to preserve the weight of the body, increases that weight, and when the food is not sufficient, and the body in consequence loses weight, tobacco restrains that loss." Hammond, *Physiological Effects of Alcohol and Tobacco*, Am. Journal of Medical Sciences, tom. XXXII. N. S., p. 319.

and sometimes diminishes the weight; and it is no less true that in each case the result is the index of heightened nutrition! This seems, of course, paradoxical. But physiology, quite as much as astronomy, is a science which is constantly obliging us to reconsider and rectify our crude off-hand conceptions.

It is by no means true that increase of the tissues in bulk and density is always a sign of improved health. We are accustomed to congratulate each other upon looking plump and rosy. But too much rosiness may be a symptom of ill-health; 'and, similarly with plumpness, there is a point beyond which obesity is a mere weariness to the spirit. Nor does a person need to become as rotund as Wouter Van Twiller in order to reach and pass this point. Many per-, sons, who are not actually corpulent, would lose weight if their nutrition could be improved. And the explanation is quite simple.

Normal nutrition is not merely the repair of tissue : it is the repair of all the tissues in the body *in due proportion*. This is a very essential qualification. Fibrous and areolar tissue, muscle, nerve, and fat are daily and hourly wasting in various degrees ; and the repair, whether great or small, must be nicely proportioned to the waste in each tissue. If a pound is added to the weight of the body, it makes all the difference in the world whether one ounce is muscle, another ounce nerve, a third ounce fat, and so on, or whether the whole pound is fat. When one tissue gets more than its fair share, the chances are that all the others must go a-begging. The co-ordinating, controlling power of the organism over its several parts is diminished,—which is the same as saying that nutrition is impaired. Evidence of this soon appears in the circumstance that the deposit of adipose tissue is no longer confined to the proper places.

Fat begins to accumulate all over the body,
in localities where little or no fat is want-
ed, and notably about the stomach and
diaphragm, causing laborious movement of
the thorax and wheezing respiration. When
a man gets into this state, it is a sign
that the ratio between the waste and the repair of his tissues has become seriously dis-
located. You can relieve him of his fat only
by improving his nutrition. The German
who drinks his forty glasses of lager bier
per diem is said to be bloated; and we
have heard it gravely surmised that the ale,
getting into his system, swells him up—as
if the human body were a sort of bladder
or balloon! The explanation is not quite
so simple. But it is easy to see how this
immense quantity of liquid, continually loading the stomach and intestines, and entailing extra labour upon all the excreting organs, should so damage the assimilative powers as to occasion an excessive deposit of

coarse fat and of flabby, imperfectly-elaborated connective tissue, over the entire surface of the body. And the state of chronic, though mild, narcosis in which the guzzler keeps himself, by still further injuring his reparative powers, contributes · to the general result.

There are consequently four ways in which tobacco may exhibit its effects upon the nutrition of the body.

I. In stimulant doses, by improving nutrition, it may increase the normal weight.

II. In stimulant doses, by improving nutrition, it may cause a diminution of weight abnormally produced.

III. In narcotic doses, by impairing nutrition, it may cause emaciation.

IV. In narcotic doses, by impairing nutrition, it may aggravate obesity instead of relieving it.[24]

---

[24] In this exposition we have assumed that the tobacco is smoked and the saliva retained. If the saliva be fre-

We may see, by this example, how much
room is always left for fallacy in the empirical tracing of physiological effects to their
causes. The phænomena are so complex that
induction is of but little avail, unless supported and confirmed by deduction.[25] In the
case of tobacco, our conclusions are so con-

---

quently ejected, the case is entirely altered. Habitual
spitting incites the salivary glands to excessive secretion,
thereby weakening the system to a surprising extent, and
probably lowering nutrition. Many temperate smokers,
who think themselves hurt by tobacco, are probably hurt
only because, though in all other respects gentlemen,
they will persist in the filthy habit of spitting. There is
no excuse for the habit, for with very little practice the
desire to get rid of the saliva entirely ceases, and is
never again felt.

In chewing, the saliva is so impregnated with the
nicotinous constituents of the leaf, that the choice
lies far more narrowly between spitting and narcosis.
Of the two evils we shall not venture to say which is
the least. In snuffing, too, the question is complicated
by the acute local irritation caused by the contact of the
stimulant with the nasal membranes. This, no doubt, has
its medicinal virtues. But for a healthy man it is probable that smoking is the only rational, as it is certainly
the only decent, way in which to use tobacco.

[25] Mill's *System of Logic*, 6th ed. vol. I. pp. 503–508.

firmed. Deduction, supported by cautious induction, shows the stimulant action of tobacco to be of permanent benefit to the system; and hence the statements of those smokers who believe themselves injured by the habit must be received with due qualifications. Yielding unsuspiciously to the influence of a prejudice which originated in an absurd puritanical notion of "morality,"[26] many smokers are in the habit of reviling the practice which they nevertheless will not abandon. Having once begun to smoke, they persist in laying to the account of tobacco sundry aches and ails which in the hurry and turmoil of modern life no one can expect wholly to escape, and many of which are such as tobacco could not possibly give rise to. If their teeth, for instance, begin to decay, tobacco gets the blame, although it is notorious to dentists that tobacco preserves

---

[26] "The Puritans, from the earliest days of their 'plantation' among us, abhorred the fume of the pipe." Fairholt, *Tobacco, its History. etc.*. p. 111.

the enamel of the teeth as hardly anything else will. We have seen teeth which had been kept for months in a preparation of nicotine and were in excellent condition. Then the headache, due perhaps to an overdose of hot risen biscuit or viands cooked in pork-fat, is quite likely to be laid to the charge of the general scape-goat; although to produce a headache directly by means of tobacco requires a powerful narcotic dose.[27]　One of the

---

[27] Smoking has also been charged with acting as a predisposing, or even as an exciting, cause of insanity,— a notion effectually disposed of by Dr. Bucknill, in the *Lancet*, Feb. 28th, 1857.

Before leaving this subject, it may be well to allude to Mr. Parton's remarks (p. 35) about "pallid," "yellow," "sickly," and "cadaverous," tobacco-manufacturers. He evidently means to convey the impression that workers in tobacco are more unhealthy than other workmen. Upon this point we shall content ourselves with transcribing the following passage from Christison, *On Poisons*, p. 731:—"Writers on the diseases of artisans have made many vague statements on the supposed baneful effects of the manufacture of snuff on the workmen. It is said they are liable to bronchitis, dysentery, ophthalmia, carbuncles, and furuncles. At a meeting of the Royal Medical Society of Paris, however, before which a memoir

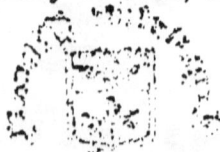

chief causes of ordinary headache is doubtless the use of the execrable anthracite which Pennsylvania protectionists force upon us by means of their unrighteous prohibitory tariff upon English coal.[23] We have even heard it alleged that smoking impairs the eyesight.

---

to this purport was lately read, the facts were contradicted by reference to the state of the workmen at the Royal Snuff Manufactory of Gros-Caillou, where 1000 people are constantly employed without detriment to their health. (*Revue Médicale*, 1827, tom. III. p. 168.) This subject has been since investigated with great care by Messrs. Parent-Duchatelet and D'Arcet, who inquired minutely into the state of the workmen employed at all the great tobacco-manufactories of France, comprising a population of above 4000 persons; and the results at which they have arrived are,—that the workmen very easily become habituated to the atmosphere of the manufactory,—that they are not particularly subject either to special diseases, or to disease generally,—and that they live on an average quite as long as other tradesmen. These facts are derived from very accurate statistical returns. (*Annales d'Hygiène*, 1829, tom. I. p. 169.)" The reader may also consult an instructive notice in Hammond's *Journal of Psychological Medicine*, Oct. 1868, vol. II. p. 828.

[28] See Dr. Derby's pamphlet on *Anthracite and Health*, Boston, 1868; and an article by the present writer, in the *World*, April 11th, 1868.

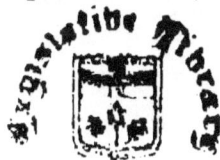

Students smoke much and are nearsighted, is the complacent argument—it being apparently forgotten that sailors smoke much and are far-sighted, and that in each case the result is due to the way in which the eyes are used.

These examples show with what well-meaning recklessness people find fault with anything which they are at all events bound to condemn. It is not to be denied, however, that many persons are continually hurting themselves by the flagrant abuse of tobacco. Many men are doubtless in a state of chronic tobacco-narcosis; just as many men and women keep themselves in a state of chronic narcosis from the abuse of tea and coffee. Probably three-fourths of the ill-health which afflicts the community is due to barbarous neglect of the plainest principles of dietetics. When a thing tickles the palate, or refreshes the nervous system, people do not seem to be as yet sufficiently civilized to let it go until they have made themselves miserable with it. Half the inhabitants of the United States, says Mr. Parton, violate the laws of nature every time they go to the dinner-table. He might safely have put the figure higher. Owing to the shortcomings of our present methods of education, we rarely get taught physiology at school or college, we never thoroughly learn the principles of hygiene, or if we acquire some of them by hearsay, we seldom realize them in such a way as to shape our behaviour accordingly. It is not to be wondered at, therefore, that people eat imprudently and smoke imprudently. They smoke just before dinner, they smoke rank, badly-cured tobacco, they smoke much, and they smoke fast, thus narcotizing instead of stimulating their nervous systems. A plum-pudding is good and nourishing, but it would hardly be wise to eat it before meat, or to eat it to the verge of nausea.

This lesson of *dosage* is one which cannot

be learned too thoroughly. The would-be reformer says, "Touch not the unclean thing;"
but the reply is, "No hurt has ever yet
come to me from smoking: I will therefore
smoke all the more, to confute these idle
crotchets." This is the very crudity of un-
disciplined inference. In physiology we cannot go by the rule of three. Doctors can
tell us how they prescribe brandy for epilepsy: exulting in his signal relief, the patient
persists in taking a second dose, and—brings
on another fit! Stimulation gives way to
narcosis. In delirium tremens the stimulus
of opium is often found to be of great service. But sometimes the unscientific physician, wishing to increase the beneficial effect,
keeps on until he has administered a narcotic dose; when lo! all is undone, the en-
feebled nerves, needing nothing but stimulus,
have received the final shock, the medulla
is paralyzed, and the heart ceases to beat.
Let no one imagine, then, that this distinc-

tion between large and small quantities is trivial or wire-drawn. In therapeutics it is often the one all-important distinction. In dealing with narcotics, it is the root of the whole matter.

And now the question arises, what *is* a stimulant dose? How much tobacco can a man take daily with benefit to himself? The reply is obvious, that no universal rule can be given. In dealing with the science of life, to indulge in sweeping statements and glittering generalities is the surest mark of a charlatan. Mr. Parton says, with reference to alcohol, that he devoutly wishes the thing could be proved to be, always, everywhere, under any circumstances, and in any quantities, injurious. (p. 59.) If this could be proved, alcohol would be shown to be a substance all but unique in nature. So much as this cannot be said of arsenic, prussic acid, or strychnine. Science cannot be made to harmonize with the exaggerations

of radicalism. With regard to tobacco, every
man, moderately endowed with common sense,
can soon tell how much he ought to take.
The muscular tremour of narcosis is unmistakable, and a depressed or fluttering pulse
is easily detected. When a man has smoked
until these symptoms are awakened, let him
stop short,—he has gone too far already.
Let him take good care never to repeat the
dose. ‾The true Epicurean, to whom μηδέν
ἄγαν has become second nature, who knows
how to live, and who is instinctively dis-
gusted by vulgar excess, will not be likely
to oversmoke himself more than once. So
much we say, in view of the impossibility of
laying down universal rules. But it is well
for the smoker to bear in mind that the
more gradually the nicotine is absorbed into
his circulating system, the better. For this
reason a pipe, with porous bowl and long
porous stem, is better than a cigar,[29] which is

---

[29] The cigar is, however, usually made of milder to

besides liable by direct contact to irritate the tongue and lips. And, likewise, it is better to smoke mild tobacco for an hour than strong tobacco for half an hour. Probably four or five pipes daily are enough for most healthy persons; but no such rule can be quoted as inflexible or infallible. Some persons, as we have said, are never stimulated by tobacco, and therefore ought never to smoke at all. Others can take relatively large quantities with little risk of narcosis. Dr. Parr would smoke twenty pipes in a single evening. The illustrious Hobbes sat always wrapped in a dense cloud of smoke, while he wrote his immortal works; yet he lived, hale and hearty, to the age of ninety-two.

We have spoken of persons who are incapable of deriving stimulus from the use of tobacco, but are always narcotized by it. We doubt if perfectly healthy persons are ever

---

bacco. And an old pipe, saturated with nicotinous oil, may become far stronger than any ordinary cigar.

4

affected in this way. In a considerable number of cases we have observed that this incapacity occurs in people who are troubled
with some chronic abnormal action or inaction
of the liver; but we have as yet been unable
to make any generalization which might serve
to connect the two phænomena. In the great
majority of cases, however, the incapacity has
been probably induced by chronic narcosis
resulting from the long-continued abuse of
tobacco. Recent researches have shown that
confirmed drunkards have after a while modi-
fied the molecular structure of their nervous
systems to such an extent that they can
never for the rest of their lives touch an alcoholic drink with safety. For such poor
creatures, teetotalism is the only hygienic
rule. It is fair to suppose that under the
continuous influence of tobacco-narcosis the
nervous system becomes metamorphosed in
some analogous manner, so that after a while
tobacco ceases to be of any use and becomes

simply noxious. This is likely to be the case with those who begin to chew or smoke when they are half-grown boys, and keep on taking enormous doses of the narcotic until they have arrived at middle age. As Mr. Parton seems to find a difficulty in realizing that any one who smokes at all can smoke less than from ten to twenty large cigars daily, (for he always uses these figures when he has occasion to allude to the subject), we presume this to be about the ration which he used to allow himself. If so, no wonder that he found it did not pay to smoke. He probably did the wisest thing he could do when he gave up the habit; and his mistake has been in endeavouring to erect the limitations of his own experience into objective laws of the universe.

To sum up the physiological argument: we have endeavoured, as precisely as possible in the present state of knowledge, to answer the question, Does it pay to smoke?, From the outset we have found it necessary to a

clear understanding of the problem to keep
steadily in mind the generic difference between the effects of tobacco when taken in
narcotic quantities and its effects when taken
in stimulant quantities. The first class of
effects we have seen to be always and necessarily bad; though not so extremely and vari-
ously bad as hygienic reformers appear to
believe.[20] With regard to the second class of
effects, we have seen reason to believe that
they are almost always good. We have seen
reason to believe that, in the first place, the
stimulant dose of tobacco retards waste; and,

---

[20] Tobacco, as we have said, may, in an adequate dose,
produce well-developed paralysis. Whether the ordinary
excessive use of it ever does cause paralysis, is, to say the
least, extremely doubtful. Dr. D. W. Cheever says, "The
minor, rarely the graver, affections of the nervous system
do follow the use of tobacco in excess. . . . . . Numerous
cases of paralysis among tobacco-takers in France were
traced to the lead in which the preparation was enveloped."
Atlantic Monthly, Aug. 1860. Another instance of the great
care needful in correctly tracing the causes of any disease
or ailment. Lead-poisoning, when chronic, brings about
structural degeneration of the nerve-centres.

in the second place, that it facilitates repair :—

I. By its action on the sympathetic ganglia, aiding digestion,—

II. By its action on the medulla oblongata, aiding the circulation,—

III. By its action on the interstitial nerve-fibres, aiding the general assimilation of prepared material.

And lastly, we have witnessed the evidence of its effect upon the increased nutrition of the brain and spinal cord, in its alleviation of abnormal wakefulness and tremour. These are legitimate scientific inferences ; and if they are to be overturned, it must be by scientific argument. They are not to be shaken by all of Mr. Parton's clamour about the Coming Man, and people who keep themselves "well-groomed," and ladies who write for the press. So far as our present knowledge of physiology goes for anything, it thus goes to exhibit tobacco, rightly used, as the great econo-

mizer of vital force, the aider of nervous
co-ordination, and one of the ablest co-work-
ers in normal and vigorous nutrition. And,
as we have said before, it is the difference in
the rate of nutrition which is probably the
most fundamental difference between strength
and feebleness, vigour and sluggishness,
health and disease. It was because of rapid
nutrition that Napoleon and Humboldt per-
formed their prodigious tasks, and yet needed
almost incredibly little sleep. It is the difference between fast and slow nutrition which
makes one soldier's wound heal, while another's
gangrenes; which enables one young girl to
throw off a chest-cold with ease, while another
is dragged into the grave by it. Waste and repair—these are the essential correlatives; and
the agent which checks the former while hasten-
ing the latter can hardly be other than a friend
to health, long life, and vigour.

We conclude with an inductive argument
which an eminent physician has recently in con-

versation urged upon our attention. Throughout the whole world, probably nine men out
of every ten use tobacco.[31] Throughout the
civilized world, women, as a general rule, ab-
stain from the use of tobacco. Here we have
an experiment, on an immense scale, ready-
made for us. These three hundred million
civilized men and women are subjected to the
same varieties of climatic, dietetic, and social
influences; their environments are the same;
their inherited organic proclivities will average
about the same; but the men smoke and the
women do not. Now, if all that our hygienic
reformers say about tobacco were true, the
men in civilized countries should be afflicted
with numerous constitutional diseases which

---

[31] Paraguay tea is used by 10,000,000 of people; coca
by 10,000,000; chicory by 40,000,000; cocoa by 50,000,000;
coffee by 100,000,000; betel by 100,000,000; haschisch
by 300,000,000; opium by 400,000,000; Chinese tea by
500,000,000; tobacco by 800,000,000; the population of the
world being probably not much over one thousand million. See Von Bibra, *Die Narkotischen Genussmittel und
der Mensch*, Preface.

do not afflict the women; or should be more
liable to the diseases common to the two
sexes; or, finally, should be shorter lived than
the women. But statistics show that men are,
on the whole, just as healthy and long-lived
as women. In point of the average number
of diseases[32] to which they are subject; in
point of liability to disease; and in point of
longevity; the two sexes are in all civilized
countries, exactly on a par with each other.
During the two hundred years in which tobacco has been in common use, it has made
no appreciable difference in the health or
longevity of those who have used it. This
is a rough experiment, in which no account is
taken of dosage, and in which the results are
only general averages. But to our mind, it is
very significant. Taken alone, it shows conclusively that since tobacco first began to be

---

[32] Omitting, of course, from the comparison, the class
of diseases to which woman is peculiarly subject, as a
child-bearer.

used, its bad effects must have been at least fully balanced by its good effects. Taken in connection with our physiological argument, it shows quite conclusively that the current notion about the banefulness of tobacco is, as we remarked above, simply a popular delusion.

To prove that tobacco, rightly used, is harmless, is to prove that it does pay to smoke. Every smoker, who has not vitiated his nervous system by raw excess, knows that there is no physical pleasure in the long run comparable with that which is afforded by tobacco. If such pleasure is to be obtained without detriment to the organism, who but the grimmest ascetic can say that here is not a gain? But, if, as we have every reason to believe, the stimulant action of tobacco upon the human system is not only harmless but very decidedly beneficial, then it is doubly proved that *it does pay to smoke.*

4*

II.

THE COMING MAN WILL DRINK WINE.

MR. PARTON treats alcohol much more re-
spectfully than he treats tobacco. Though
equally hostile to it, he apparently considers
it a more formidable enemy. Instead of taking for granted from the outset that which it
is his business to prove, he now condescends
to employ something which to the unpractised
eye may look like scientific argument. He
has taken pains to collect such evidence as
may be made to support his view of the case.
And he frequently endeavours to assume an
attitude of apparent impartiality by alluding
to himself as a drinker of " these seductive
liquids,"—although, in point of fact, his whole
essay is conceived in the narrowest spirit of
radical teetotalism. As for tobacco, it does

not seem to occur to him that any one can be
found, so obstinate or so deluded as seriously to
maintain that there is any good in it; and he
therefore writes upon that subject with all the
exaggeration of unterrified confidence. But in
dealing with alcohol, his violence of statement
is evidently due to an uneasy consciousness
that there is a vast body of current opinion
and of scientific doctrine which may be arrayed
in the lists against him. He brushes away,
with a contemptuous sneer, (p. 56) the opinions
of the medical profession; but he is, nevertheless, unable wholly to ignore them. Propositions of the sort which he formerly alluded to
as if no one could think of doubting them, he
now thinks it necessary to state at length.
The poisonous nature of tobacco could be taken
for granted in a subordinate clause; but the
poisonous nature of alcohol needs to be asserted
in an independent sentence. "Pure alcohol,
though a product of highly nutritive substances,
is a mere poison,—an absolute poison,—the

mortal foe of life in every one of its forms, animal and vegetable." (p. 64.)

This is the way in which the advocates of total abstinence like to begin. A good round assertion about "poison" is calculated to demoralize the inexperienced reader, and to scare him into half giving up the case at once. But it is not all barking dogs that bite. 'Morphia is a deadly poison; but opium, which contains it, is not "the mortal foe of life in all its forms,"—it is sometimes the only thing which will keep soul and body together.[1] Theine is no doubt a deadly poison, but we manage to drink it with tolerable safety in our tea and coffee. Lactucin is probably a poison, yet people may eat a lettuce-salad and live. Chlorine is eminently a poison, yet we are all the

---

[1] Opium, as used in moderation by Orientals, has not been proved to exercise any deleterious effects. Very likely it is a healthful stimulant; but it does not appear to agree with the constitutions of the Western races. See Pharmaceutical Journal, vol. xi. p. 364. Probably tea, tobacco and alcohol are the only stimulants adapted alike to all races, and to nearly all kinds of people.

time taking it into our systems, combined with sodium, in the shape of table-salt. Therefore over the verbal question whether a teaspoonful of pure alcohol is a poison, we do not care to wrangle. People do not drink pure alcohol, as a general thing. And as for the beverages into the composition of which alcohol enters, the reader will have no difficulty in understanding that they are poisons in just the same sense in which common salt and oxygen are poisons; *i. e.*, if you take enough of them, they will kill you. This point was sufficiently cleared up in our first chapter.

Mr. Parton's hostility to this " mortal foe of life in all its forms" has taken shape in six definite propositions. Concerning alcoholic liquor of any kind and in any quantity, he asserts, and attempts to prove, that it does not nourish, that it does not aid digestion, that it does not warm, that it does not strengthen, that it undergoes no chemical change in the system, and that it always injuriously affects

' the brain. Beginning with the last of these propositions, let us first see what Mr. Parton has to say for it.

"If I, at this ten A. M., full of interest in this subject, and eager to get my view of it upon paper, were to drink a glass of the best port, Madeira, or sherry, or even a glass of lager-bier, I should lose the power to continue in three minutes; or, if I persisted in going on, I should be pretty sure to utter paradox and spurts of extravagance, which would not bear the cold review of to-morrow morning. Any one can try this experiment. Take two glasses of wine, and then immediately apply yourself to the hardest task your mind ever has to perform, and you will find you cannot do it. Let any student, just before he sits down to his mathematics, drink a pint of the purest beer, and he will be painfully conscious of loss of power." Did it ever dimly occur to Mr. Parton that all men may not be constructed on exactly the same plan with himself?

We wonder how many drops of "seductive fluid," unwisely taken at the wrong time of day, are to be held responsible for the following "spurt" of extravagance: "The time, I hope, is at hand, when an audience in a theatre, who catch a manager cheating them out of their fair allowance of fresh air, will not sit and gasp, and inhale destruction till eleven P. M., and then rush wildly to the street for relief. They will stop the play; they will tear up the benches, if necessary; they will throw things on the stage; they will knock a hole in the wall; they will *have* the means of breathing, or perish in the struggle." Is this the way in which "well-groomed" people are expected to behave? Fancy an audience following this precious bit of advice. When Mlle. Janauschek, for instance, is finishing the third act of "Medea" or the second act of "Deborah," amid the tragic solemnity of the scene, fancy the audience, because of bad

air in the theatre, getting up and flinging
their canes and opera-glasses on the stage,
in the heroic struggle for oxygen or death!
Fancy four or five hundred grown-up, educated people behaving in this way! If these
are to be the manners of the Coming Man,
we trust it will be long before he comes.

Such is one of the "spurts of extravagance" which Mr. Parton apparently thinks
will "bear the cold review of to-morrow
morning." Having survived this, we may
philosophically resign ourselves to the in-
fliction of another, more nearly akin to our
subject. "How we all wondered that England should *think* so erroneously, and adhere
to its errors so obstinately, during our late
war! Mr. Gladstone has in part explained
the mystery. The adults of England, he
said, in his famous wine-speech, drink, on an
average, three hundred quarts of beer each
per annum!" Another choice bit of radical
philosophy: if your neighbour happens not

to agree with your most cherished opinions,
he must be idiotic, immoral, or *drugged!*
The English failed to sympathize with us,
because they are such beer-drinkers! What
a rare faculty of disentangling causal rela-
tions! We believe that the working people,
who drink the most beer, were just those
who, as a class, were most ready to sympathize with us in the time of need. But
Mr. Parton has "grounds" for his opinion.
"It is physically impossible for a human
brain, muddled every day with a quart of
beer, to correctly hold correct opinions, or
appropriate pure knowledge." "The recep-
tive, the curious, the candid, the trustworthy
brains,—those that do not take things for
granted, and yet are ever open to convic-
tion,—such heads are to be found on the
shoulders of men who drink little or none
of these seductive fluids." Mr. Parton has
doubtless forgotten that the head of "the
nearest approach to the complete human

being that has yet appeared," the head of
the "highly-groomed" Goethe—rested upon
the shoulders of a man who drank his two
or three bottles of wine daily.[2] But we
are now rapidly getting into the æthereal
region of certainties. "Taking together all
that science and observation teach and in-
dicate, we have one certainty: that, to a
person in good health and of good life,
alcoholic liquors are not necessary, but are
always in some degree hurtful." So it is
not an open question, after all! Certainty
has been arrived at, — by Mr. Parton, at
least. And it is so difficult to suppose that
any sane mind, after due investigation, can
come to a different opinion, that all persons
who mean to keep on using alcohol are
advised in pathetic language never to look
into the facts:

"If ignorance is bliss, 't is folly to be wise."

The candid reader must admit that Mr.

[2] Lewes, *Life of Goethe*, vol. II. p. 267.

Parton has not, so far, made out a very overwhelming case in support of his opinion that alcohol always injures the brain. A personal experience, a "spurt of extravagance," a "physical impossibility," and a "certainty," are, on the whole, not very rocky foundations upon which to build a scientific conclusion. But this is all Mr. Parton has to offer.

In attempting to describe the influence of alcohol upon the brain and nervous system, it will be well for us to keep steadily in mind the fundamental difference between stimulant and narcotic doses, which was described at some length in our chapter on Tobacco. It is hardly necessary to state that Mr. Parton neither recognizes, nor appears dimly to suspect, the existence of any such distinction. His is one of those minds in which there are no half-way stations. With him, to rise above zero is inevitably to fly to the boiling-water point. But with-

out keeping in mind this all-important distinction, any inquiry into the physiological
effects of alcohol must end in confusion and
paradox. Remembering this, let us examine
first the narcotic, and then the stimulant
effects of alcohol upon the nervous system.

The narcotic effects of alcohol upon the
entire human organism are so bad that
even the teetotaler does not need to exag-
gerate them. The stomach is not only dam-
aged, and the cerebrum ruined, but a slow
molecular change takes place throughout the
nervous system, which ends by destroying
the power of self-control and utterly demoralizing the character. Far be it from us,
therefore, to palliate the consequences which
sooner or later are sure to follow the
wretched habit of drinking narcotic quantities
of alcohol; or to look without genuine sympathy upon the philanthropic, though usually
misguided attempts which radical aquarians
are continually making to diminish the evil.

Their feelings are often as right as their science is wrong. But because we believe that for a book to be of any value whatever, it must be *true*, and that false science can never, in the long run, be of practical benefit, we are not therefore to be set down as lukewarm in our abhorrence of alcoholic intemperance. Those who keep their hearts in subjection to their heads are often supposed to have no hearts at all. Those who do not forthwith get angry and utter "spurts of extravagance" whenever any social evil is mentioned, are often thought to be in secret sympathy with it. But how could we, by writing reams of fervid declamation, more forcibly express our disapproval of drunkenness than by recording the cold scientific statement that the first narcotic symptom produced by alcohol is a symptom of incipient paralysis?

We allude to the flushing of the face, which is caused by paralysis of the cervical

branch of the sympathetic. This symptom
usually occurs some time before the conspicuous manifestation of the ordinary signs of intoxication, which result from paralysis of the
cerebrum. Of these signs the most prominent
is the weakening of the ordinary power of self-
control. The ruling faculty of judgment is
suspended, volition becomes less steady, and
imagination, no longer guided by the higher
faculties, runs riot in such a way as to appear to be stimulated. But it is not stimulated; it is simply let loose. There is no
stimulation in drunkenness; there is only disorganization. One acquired or organic power
of the mind no longer holds the others in
check. Hence the uncalled-for friendliness,
the fitful anger, the extravagant or misplaced
generosity, the ludicrous dignity, the disgusting amorousness, or the garrulous vanity, of
the drunken man. Wine is said to exhibit a
man as he really is, with the conventionalities
of society laid aside. This is only half true,

but it suggests the true statement. Wine exhibits a man as he is when the organized effects of ancestral and contemporary civilization upon his character are temporarily obliterated. We need no better illustration of the truth that drunkenness is not stimulation but paralysis of the cerebrum, than the order in which, under the influence of alcohol, the powers of the mind become progressively suspended. As a general rule those are first suspended which are the most recent products of civilization, and which have consequently been developed by inheritance through the least number of generations. These are of course the mind's highest organic acquisitions. The sense of responsibility, for instance, is a product of a highly complicated state of civilization, and, when fully developed, is perhaps chief among the moral acquirements which distinguish the civilized man from the savage. In progressing intoxication, the feeling of responsibility is the first to be put in abeyance.

A man need be but slightly tipsy in order to become quite careless as to the consequences of his actions.[3]   On the other hand, those qualities of the mind are the last to be overcome, which are the earliest inheritance of savagery, and which the civilized man possesses in common with savages and beasts. Then the animal nature of the man, no longer restrained by his higher faculties, manifests itself with a violence which causes it to seem abnormally stimulated in vigour. And in the stage immediately preceding stupor, it sometimes happens that the pupils are contracted,[4] and the whites of the eyes enlarged, giving to the face a horrible brute-like expression.

---

[3] In illustration it may be noted that as soon as a man has just transgressed the physiological limit which divides stimulation from narcosis, he is liable to throw overboard all prudential considerations and drink until he is completely drunk. This is one of the chief dangers of convivial after-dinner drinking.

[4] For the physiology of this pupil-change, not uncommon in various kinds of acute narcosis, see the Appendix to Anstie.

One apparent exception to this generalization needs only to be explained in order to confirm the rule. Memory, which usually figures as a high intellectual faculty, is often, even in deep drunkenness, capable of performing marvellous feats. While in college we once heard a tipsy fellow-student repeat *verbatim* the whole of that satire of Horace which begins "Unde et quo, Catius?"—which he had read over the same day before going to recitation, but which, as we felt sure, he could never designedly have committed to memory. It appeared, however, that, in the literal though not in the idiomatic sense of the phrase, he had "committed it to memory" to some purpose, for as we, struck with amazement, took down our Horace and followed him, we found that he made not the slightest verbal error. This performance on his part was almost immediately followed by heavy comatose slumber. On afterward questioning him, it appeared that he remembered

5

nothing either of the Satire or of his remarkable feat. Several analogous cases are cited by Dr. Anstie.[5]

This certainly looks like stimulation, but on comparing it with other instances of abnormal reminiscence differently caused, we shall find reason for believing that it is nothing of the kind. There is no doubt that insanity may in the most general way be described as a species of cerebral paralysis, yet in many kinds of insanity there is an abnormal quickening of memory. Likewise in idiocy, which differs from insanity as being due to arrested development rather than to degradation of the cerebrum, the same phænomenon is sometimes witnessed. We remember seeing a child who, though generally considered quite " foolish," could, as we were assured, accurately repeat large portions of each Sunday's sermon. Dr. Anstie mentions a boy, absolutely idiotic, who nevertheless " had a perfect

---

[5] *Stimulants and Narcotics*, pp. 174–178.

memory for the history of all the farm animals in the neighbourhood, and could tell with unerring precision that this was So-and-so's sheep or pig among any number of other animals of the same kind." Similar phænomena have been observed in epileptic delirium, and in the delirium of fevers. Every one has heard Coleridge's story of the sick servant-girl who repeated passages from Latin, Greek and Hebrew authors which she had years before heard recited by a clergyman in whose house she worked. A gentleman in India, after a sunstroke, utterly lost his command of the Hindustani language, recovering it only during the recurrent paroxysms of epileptic delirium to which he was afterward subject. Equally interesting is the case of the Countess de Laval, who in the ravings of puerperal delirium was heard by her Breton nurse talking baby-talk to herself in the Breton language,— a language which she had known in early infancy, but had since so entirely forgotten as

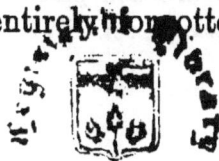

not to distinguish it from gibberish when spoken before her.[6] A similar exaltation of memory not unfrequently precedes the coma produced by chloroform ; and it has been known to occur in cases of acute poisoning by opium and haschisch. Finally it may be observed that drowning men are said to recall, as in a panoramic vision, all the events of their lives, even the most trivial.

We may conclude therefore that the extraordinary memory sometimes observed in drunken persons, however obscure the interpretation of it may at present be, is at all events a symptom, not of mental exaltation, but of mental disorganization consequent upon cerebral disease. We may search in vain among the phænomena of intoxication for any genuine evidences of that heightened mental activity which is said to be followed by a depressive recoil. There is no recoil;

[6] For this and parallel cases see Hamilton, *Lectures on Metaphysics*, Lect. XVIII.

there is no stimulation; there is nothing but paralytic disorder from the moment that narcosis begins. From the outset the whole nervous system is lowered in tone, the even course of its nutrition disturbed, and the rhythmic discharge of its functions interfered with.

Another remarkable effect of alcoholic narcotism—the most hopelessly demoralizing of all—yet remains to be treated. We refer to the perpetual craving of the drinker for the repetition, and usually for the increase, of his dose. It is a familiar fact that the drunkard is urged to the gratification of his appetite by such an irresistible physical craving that his power of self-control becomes after a while completely destroyed. And it is often observed that those who begin drinking moderately go on, as if by a kind of fatality, drinking oftener and drinking larger quantities, until they have become confirmed inebriates. But in the current interpretation of these facts there is, as might be expected, a great deal of confusion. On the one hand, the teetotalers declare that the use of alcohol in any amount creates a physical craving and necessitates a progressive increase of the dose. On the other hand, the common sense of mankind, perceiving that nine persons out of ten are all their lives in the habit of using alcoholic drinks, while hardly one person out of ten ever becomes a drunkard,[1] declares that this physical craving is not produced save in peculiarly organized constitutions. We be-

---

[1] It has been asserted by teetotalers that the mortality from intemperance is 50,000 a year in the United States alone!! It is to be regretted that friends of temperance are to be found who will persist in injuring the cause by such wanton exaggerations. In the United States, in 1860, the whole number of deaths from all causes was a trifle less than 374,000: the whole number of deaths from intemperance was 931,—that is to say, less than one in 374. See the admirable pamphlet by the late Gov. Andrew, on *The Errors of Prohibition*, p. 112. In view of these facts, it appears to us many leagues within the bounds of probability to say that hardly one person in ten is a drunkard.

lieve that neither of these opinions is correct. In all probability, the demand for an increased narcotic effect is due to a gradual alteration in the molecular structure of the nervous system caused by frequently repeated narcosis; and if narcosis be invariably avoided, *in systems which are free from its inherited structural effects*, the craving is never awakened. This point is so interesting and important as to call for some further elucidation.

Frequent intoxication with alcohol, opium, coca, or haschisch, brings about a structural degeneration of the nerve-material; the consequences of which are to be seen in delirium, softening of the brain, and other forms of general paralysis. "By degrees the nervous centres, especially those on which the particular narcotic used has the most powerful influence, become degraded in structure." A permanent pathological state is thus induced, in which the production of a given narcotic effect is not so easy as in the healthy organism. "A certain quantity of nervous tissue has in fact ceased to fill the *rôle* of nervous tissue, and there is less of impressible matter upon which the narcotic may operate, and hence it is that the confirmed drunkard, opium-eater, or *coquero*, requires more and more of his accustomed narcotic to produce the intoxication which he delights in. It is necessary now to saturate his blood to a high degree with the poison, and thus to insure an extensive contact of it with the nervous matter, if he is to enjoy once more the transition from the realities of life to the dreamland, or the pleasant vacuity of mind, which this or the other form of narcotism has hitherto afforded him."[8] It is easy to see how this structural degeneration may be produced. It takes a certain time for the nervous system to recover from the effects of each separate narcotic dose; and if a fresh dose is taken

---

[8] See Anstie, op. cit. pp. 215, 216, 218.

before recovery is completed, it is obvious that the diseased condition will by and by be rendered permanent. The entire process of nutrition will adapt itself gradually to this new state of things; and no efficiency of repair will afterward make the nervous system what it was before. It is in this way that the narcotic craving for continually increased doses is originated and kept alive.

In the case of the milder narcotics—tea, coffee and tobacco—this craving, though the symptom of a depraved state of the organism, does not directly demoralize the character. But the moral injury wrought by alcohol, opium and haschisch is known to every one, and the effects of coca-drunkenness are said to be no less frightful. This is because the milder narcotics affect chiefly the medulla, the spinal cord and the sympathetic, while the fiercer ones chiefly affect the cerebrum. Tobacco may paralyze the brain sufficiently to cause nocturnal wakefulness; but it can-

5*

not impair one's self-control or one's sense
of responsibility. It never transforms a man
into a selfish brute, who will beat his wife,
neglect his business, and allow his children
to starve. Here then we arrive at a su-
premely interesting distinction. The craving
for tobacco is principally a craving of those
inferior nerve-centres which exert compara-
tively little direct influence upon the mental
and moral life. But the craving for alcohol
is a cerebral craving. The habitual in-
dulgence of it involves a continual sup-
pression of those loftier guiding qualities
which, as we have seen, are the later effects
of civilization upon the individual character;
while the attributes of savagery, the lower
sensual passions—our common inheritance
from pre-social times—are allowed full play
in supplying material for the imagination
and in shaping the purposes of life. Mr.
Parton's remark, therefore, which is absurd
as applied to tobacco, is a profound physi-

ological verity as applied to the narcotic action of alcohol,—it tends to make us think and act like barbarians, for it allies us psychologically with barbarians.

These considerations throw some light upon the way in which chronic narcosis, like other diseases entailing structural derangements, may be transmitted from father to son. As a matter of observation it is known that drunkenness may run· through whole families, no less than gout or consumption. Or, like other diseases, it may skip one or two generations and then reappear. It is evident that the children of a drunkard, *born after* the establishment of nervous degeneration in the father's system, may inherit structural narcosis attended by a latent craving for alcohol. Some unfortunate persons thus seem to be born sots, as others are born lunatics or consumptives.

The hygienic rule in all cases of structural narcosis, whether acquired or inherited,

is total abstinence once and always. These
unfortunate creatures cannot be temperate,
they must therefore be abstinent. As Sainte-
Beuve profoundly remarks concerning that
ferocious Duke of Burgundy for whom Fé-
nelon wrote his "Télémaque," he was such a
wretch that they could not make a *man* of
him, they could only make him a *saint:*
that is, he was got up on such wrong principles that, whether bad or good, he must
be somewhat morally lop-sided and abnormal. Just so with those whose nervous
systems are impaired by alcohol: we cannot
make them healthy men who can take a
stimulant glass and want no more,—we can
only make them teetotalers.

Those too who have not got themselves
into this predicament will do well to remember that there is extreme danger in the
common practice of drinking as much as
one likes, provided one does not get drunk.
"Getting drunk" means paralysis of the cer-

ebral hemispheres; but, as we have seen,
paralysis of the cervical sympathetic, shown
in flushed face and moist forehead, occurs
some time before the more conspicuous
symptom. *It is a narcotic effect, and must
be always avoided, if the narcotic craving is
to be kept clear of.* Therefore a man who
wishes to enjoy alcohol, and reap benefit
from it, and be ready at any time to do
without it, like any other wholesome aliment, must always keep a long way this
side of intoxication. If ten glasses of sherry
will make him garrulous, he will do well
never to drink more than four.

Before leaving this part of the subject,
it may be well to note certain cases, col-
lected by Theodore Parker, of consumptive
families, in which those members who were
topers did not die of consumption. It appeared that, in certain families whose his-
tories he gave, nearly all those who did not
die of consumption were rum-drinkers! And

4*

from these data Mr. Parker drew the inference that "intemperate habits (where the
man drinks a pure, though coarse and fiery
liquor like New England Rum) tend to check
the consumptive tendency, though the drunkard, who himself escapes the consequences,
may transmit the fatal seed to his children."
Mr. Parton, who quotes this, thinks it poor
comfort for topers. We doubt if there is
any "comfort" to be found in it. It is contrary to all our present science to suppose
that consumption can be prevented by narcosis. The prime cause of consumption is
defective assimilation: the tissues, *from lack
of sufficient nerve-stimulus*, are incapable of
appropriating food. How absurd, therefore,
to suppose that narcosis, which impairs the
stimulating energy of the nerves, can check an
existing tendency to consumption! What the
consumptive person needs is stimulus, not paralysis. But it is easy to believe that the same
impaired nutrition of the nerves which may

in one person end in consumption, may in
another person act as a predisposing cause
of narcosis. Insanity, consumption, and
drunkenness, are diseases which appear to
go hand in hand. Dr. Maudsley, in his
great work on the "Pathology of Mind,"
gives instructive tables which show that
these three diseases may alternate with each
other in the same family for several generations, culminating finally in epilepsy, idiocy,
paralysis and impotence, when the family
becomes happily extinct. This consanguinity
of diseases appears more marked when we
extend our view over a certain extensive
locality. The figures cited by Gov. Andrew
appear to show that both drunkenness and
insanity are far more common in New England than in other parts of the Union; and
consumption is proverbially the New England
disease. We are inclined to suspect, therefore, that in the families mentioned by Mr.
Parker, the children inherited structurally

defective nervous systems, the consequent symptoms being in one case pulmonary and in another case cerebral.

This, we believe, is all that we need contribute at present to the subject of alcoholic narcosis. It will be seen that in maintaining that the Coming Man will drink wine, we are not recommending that the Coming Man should go to bed drunk. An argument drawn from purely scientific data, when once thoroughly mastered, is likely to be of more avail in checking intemperance than all the "spurts of extravagance" which teetotalers can emit between now and doomsday. Mr. Parton asks, Why have the teetotalers failed? They have failed because they have exaggerated. They have failed because they have not been content with the simple truth. They want the truth, the whole truth, and twice as much as the truth. If they would only hoard up the nervous energy which they expend in making a vain clamour, in order to use it in quietly investigating the character, causes, and conditions of alcoholic drunkenness, they might make out a statement which the world would believe, and by and by act upon. At present the world does not follow them, because it does not believe them. When the zealous aquarian anathematizes a rum-shop, we sympathize with him; but when he rolls up his eyes in holy horror at a glass of lager-bier, we laugh at him. When he says that a quart of raw gin taken at a couple of gulps will kill a man stone-dead, we cheerfully acquiesce. But when he says that the gill of sherry taken at dinner will impair our digestion, render us susceptible to cold, steal away some of our vigour, and muddle our head so that we cannot write an article in the evening,—we can but good-naturedly smile, and try another gill to-morrow.

The stimulant effects of alcohol upon the nervous system are very similar to those of tobacco. Like tobacco, alcohol stimulates the alimentary secretions, slightly quickens and strengthens the pulse, diminishes weariness, cures sleeplessness, puts an end to trembling, calms nervous excitement, retards waste, and facilitates repair. By its antiparalytic action, it checks epilepsy, quiets delirium, and alleviates spasms and clonic convulsions; and in typhoid fever, where excessive waste of the nervous system is supposed to be one of the chief sources of danger, it is used, as we shall presently see, with most signal success. It thus appears, like tobacco, to be in general an economizer of vital energy and an aid to effective nutrition. It also directly assists digestion; but as Mr. Parton thinks it does not do this, we will first quote his opinion, and then see how much it is worth.

"Several experiments have been made with a view to ascertain whether mixing alcohol with the gastric juice increases or lessens its power to decompose food, and the results

of all of them point to the conclusion that
the alcohol retards the process of decomposition. A little alcohol retards it a little, and
much alcohol retards it much. It has been
proved by repeated experiment that *any* portion of alcohol, however small, diminishes the
power of the gastric juice to decompose. The
digestive fluid has been mixed with wine,
beer, whisky, brandy, and alcohol diluted with
water, and kept at the temperature of the
living body, and the motions of the body imi-
tated during the experiment; but, in every
instance, the pure gastric juice was found to
be the true and sole digester, and the alcohol
a retarder of digestion. This fact, however,
required little proof. We are all familiar with
alcohol as a *preserver*, and scarcely need to
be reminded that, if alcohol assists digestion
at all, it cannot be by assisting decomposition." (p. 64.)

We would give something to know how
many readers, outside of the medical profes-

sion, may have detected at the first glance
the fatal fallacy lurking in this argument. Of
its existence Mr. Parton himself is blissfully
unconscious. The experiment, no doubt, seems
quite complete and conclusive. We have the
gastric juice mixed with alcoholic liquor, we
have the suitable temperature, and we have
an imitation of the motions of the stomach.
What more can be desired? We reply, the
most important element in the problem is entirely overlooked. It is the old story,—the
play of Hamlet with the part of Hamlet left
out; and nothing can better illustrate the
extreme danger of reasoning confidently from
what goes on outside the body to what must
go on inside the body. For in order to have
made their experiment complete, Mr. Parton's
authorities *should have manufactured an entire
nervous system,* as well as a network of blood-
vessels through which the alcohol might im-
part to that nervous system its stimulus. In
short, before we can make an artificial di-

gestive apparatus which will work at all like
.the natural one, we must know how to con-
struct a living human body! In the case before us, *the nervous stimulus*, ignored by Mr. Parton, is the most essential factor in the whole
process. There is no doubt that a given
quantity of undiluted gastric juice will usually
perform the chemical process of food-trans-
formation more rapidly than an equal quantity of gastric juice which is diluted.[9] But
there is also no doubt that when we take a
small quantity of alcohol into the stomach,
the amount of gastric juice is instantly increased.
This results from the stimulant action of alcohol both upon the pneumogastric nerves and
upon the great splanchnic or visceral branches
of the sympathetic. Just as when tobacco is
smoked, though probably to a less extent, the

---

[9] This is not always true, however: it is well to look
sharp before making a sweeping statement. The digesting power of gastric juice is *increased* by diluting it
with a certain amount of water. See Lehmann, *Physio-
logische Chemie,* II. 47.

gastric secretion is increased; and the motions
of the stomach are also increased. This increase in the quantity of the digestive fluid,
due to nervous stimulus, is undoubtedly more
than sufficient to make up for the alleged
impairment of its quality caused by mixing
it with a foreign substance. The action of
saliva and carbonate of soda supply us with
a further illustration. In artificial experiments, like those upon which Mr. Parton relies, alkaline substances are found to retard
digestion by neutralizing a portion of the acid
of the gastric juice. Yet the alkaline saliva,
swallowed with food, does not retard digestion; and Claude Bernard has shown that
carbonate of soda actually hastens, to a notable degree, the digestive process. Why is
this? It is because these alkalies act as
local stimulants upon the lining of the stomach, and thus increase the quantity of gastric
juice. It is in this way that common salt,
eaten with other food, also facilitates diges-

tion; although salt is a *preserver*, as well as alcohol.

Here we come upon Mr. Parton's second blunder. He talks about the "decomposition" of food, and appears to think that digestion is a kind of *putrefaction,* so that alcohol, which arrests the latter, must also arrest the former. He says: We do not need to experiment, for we *know* that alcohol, which is a *preserver,* cannot digest food by decomposing it. This unlucky remark illustrates the danger of writing on a subject, the rudiments of which you have not taken time to get acquainted with. Before attempting to lay down the law upon an abstruse point connected with the subject of digestion, common prudence would appear to dictate that one should first acquire some dim notion of what digestion is. The veriest tyro in physiology should know that the gastric juice is itself a preventer of putrefaction. It will not only keep off organic decay, but it will stop it after

it has begun.[10]   In this sense of the word,
it is as much a *preserver* as alcohol.

As it takes time to expose all the fallacies
which Mr. Parton can crowd into one short
paragraph, we have thus far admitted that
alcohol impairs the quality of the gastric juice
by diluting it: as a matter of fact, it does
not so impair it.   If it is a *preserver*, it is
also a *coagulator*.   It coagulates the albu-
minous portions of the food, thus enabling
them to be more easily acted upon by the
gastric secretion.[11]   So that, on looking into
the matter, we find the stimulant dose of alcohol doing everything to quicken, and nothing
whatever to slacken, digestion.   It coaxes out
more digestive fluid, and it lightens the task
which that fluid has to perform.

Daily experience tells us that the glass of
wine taken with our dinner, or the thimble-

---

[10] Dunglison, *Human Physiology*, vol. I. p. 148; Lewes,
Physiology of Common Life, vol. I. p. 170.

[11] Dunglison, op. cit. I. 196.

full of *liqueur* taken after dessert, diminishes the feeling of heaviness, and enables us sooner to go to work. Of indigestion and its accompanying sensations, we are unable to speak from experience ; but Mr. Parton feelingly describes the effects of alcohol as follows. "When we have taken too much shad for breakfast, we find that a wineglass of whisky instantly mitigates the horrors of indigestion, and enables us again to contemplate the future without dismay." Now, if Mr. Parton's ideas on this subject were correct, his dose of whisky ought to exasperate his torment. The fact that it'comforts him shows that it serves to quicken the too sluggish stomach to its normal activity. It is a very good clinical experiment indeed.

Alcohol, however, aids digestion only when taken in moderate quantities. A narcotic dose, by paralyzing the medulla and the sympathetic, interferes with the flow of gas-

tric juice. Here, as in most cases, the large
quantity does just the reverse of what the
small quantity will do. The same is true
of food. Digestible food, in moderate amount,
stimulates the gastric secretion; in excessive
amount, it arrests its action. "Another curious fact is, that although the addition of
organic acids increases the digestive power
of this fluid, there is a limit at which this
increase ceases, and beyond it, excess of
acid suspends the whole digestive power."[12]
It is therefore a wise thing to eat heartily,
but a silly thing to eat voraciously; it is
wise to eat pickles, but silly to make one's
dinner of them; it is wise to drink a glass
of sherry, but silly to empty the bottle.
The happy mean is the thing to be maintained, in digestion as in every thing else.

Mr. Parton next proceeds to deny that
alcohol is a heat-producing substance. "On
the contrary," he says, "it appears in all

[12] Lewes, loc. cit.

cases to diminish the efficiency of the heat-
producing process." And he cites the testimony of Arctic voyagers, New York car-
drivers, Russian corporals, and Rocky Moun-
tain hunters, in support of the statement
that alcohol diminishes the power of the
system to resist cold. He thinks he could
fill a whole magazine with the evidence on
this point. Nevertheless, so far as we have
examined the reports of Arctic travellers,[13]
they appear by no means decisive. They
do not keep in mind the distinction between
stimulation and intoxication. We do not
doubt that "men who start under the influence of liquor are the first to succumb to
the cold, and the likeliest to be frost-bit-
ten," if the phrase "under the influence of
liquor" be understood, as it usually is, to
mean "partly drunk." On the other hand,
it is a familiar fact that a glass of whis-

---

[13] A good summary will be found in the *American
Journal of Medical Sciences*, July, 1859.

ky, taken on coming into the house after
exposure to cold, will in many cases prevent sore throat or inflammation of the
nasal passages. In our own experience, we
know of no more efficient agent for remov-
ing the effects of a chill from the system.
Before this question can be settled, however,
we must ascertain whether alcohol is, or is
not, a true food. If the food-action of alcohol is, as Liebig maintains, to be ranked
with that of fat, starch and sugar, its heat-
producing power will follow as an inevitable
inference. To this point we shall presently
come; and meanwhile we may content ourselves with citing the excellent authority of
Johnston in support of the opinion that
ardent spirits "directly warm the body." [14]

Mr. Parton next indicts alcohol on the
ground that it is not a strength-giver. "On
this branch of the subject," he observes,

---

[14] *Chemistry of Common Life*, vol. I., p. 288.

" *all* the testimony is against alcoholic drinks."[15] Yet in his own statement of the case may be found contradictions enough. On the one hand he cites Tom Sayers, Richard Cobden and Benjamin Franklin in support of his opinion;[16] and he tells us how Horace Greeley, teetotaler, coming home the other day, and finding terrible arrears of work piled up before him, sat down and wrote steadily, without leaving his room, from ten A. M. till eleven P. M.—no very wonderful feat for a healthy man. But on the other hand, it appears from some of his own facts that when a supreme exertion of strength is requisite, then we must take alcohol.

---

[15] Except that of contemporary physiologists. Among these there are few greater names than that of Moleschott; whose testimony to the strengthening properties of alcohol may be found in his *Lehre der Nahrungsmittel*, p. 162.

[16] We presume Mr. Parton thinks these three unprofessional opinions enough to outweigh the all but unanimous testimony of physicians to the tonic effects of beer wine and brandy.

"During the war I knew of a party of cavalry who, for three days and three nights, were not out of the saddle fifteen minutes at a time. The men consumed two quarts of whisky each, and all of them came in alive. It is a custom in England to extract the last possible five miles from a tired horse, when those miles *must* be had from him, by forcing down his most unwilling throat a quart of beer." (p. 86.) From these unwelcome facts Mr. Parton draws the sage inference that alcohol, like tobacco, supports us in doing wrong! "It enables us to violate the laws of nature without immediate suffering and speedy destruction." Now there is one much abused faculty of mankind, which nevertheless will sometimes refuse to be insulted,—that faculty is common sense. And in the present case, common sense declares that when we are taxing our strength, no matter whether "laws" are violated or

not, we do not keep ourselves up by drinking a substance which can only weaken us.
It may be unfortunate that alcohol is a
strength - giver; but the fact that we can
travel farther with it than without it shows
that, unfortunate or not, the thing is so. But
Mr. Parton believes that Nature is even
with us afterward. " In a few instances of
intermittent disease, a small quantity of wine
may sometimes enable a patient who is at
the low tide of vitality to anticipate the turn
of the tide, and borrow at four o'clock enough
of five o'clock strength to enable him to
reach five o'clock." This is sheer nonsense.
There is no such thing as borrowing at four
o'clock the strength of five o'clock. The
thing is a physiological absurdity. The strength
of to-morrow is non-existent until to-morrow
comes; it is not a reserved fund from which
we can borrow to-day. If Mr. Parton's notion were correct, his patient ought to be

weaker at five o'clock by just the same amount that he is stronger at four o'clock. If the strength has been borrowed, it cannot be used over again. You cannot eat your cake and save it. In an hour's time, therefore, the patient should be weaker than if he had contrived to get along without the wine. But this is not found to be the case: he is stronger at four and he is stronger at five, he is stronger next day, and he convalesces more rapidly than if he had not taken alcohol. This is a clinical fact which there is no blinking.[17] It shows that the only source from which the strength can possibly come is the alcohol. Whether it be food or not, the action of alcohol in these cases is precisely similar to that of food. It calms delirium and promotes refreshing sleep, exactly like a meat broth, except that it is often more rapidly efficient. It can produce these effects only by acting as a genuine stimulant, by either

---

[17] Anstie, op. cit. pp. 381—385.

nourishing, or facilitating the normal nutrition of, the nervous system.[18]

When therefore Lawyer Heavy-fee and the other allegorical personages mentioned by Mr. Parton sit up working all night, and then quiet their nerves by a glass of wine or a cigar, they are no doubt shortening their lives and committing "respectable suicide." But it is because they sit up all night and waste vital force, not because they resort to an obvious and effective means of repairing the loss. It is well to keep early hours and avoid overwork. But on rare occasions, when the circumstances of life absolutely require it, he who cannot sit up all night for a week together, without inflicting permanent injury

---

[18] In view of these and similar facts, Dr. Anstie remarks that "the effect of nutritious food, where it can be digested, is undistinguishable from that of alcohol upon the abnormal conditions of the nervous system which prevail in febrile diseases." p. 385. For the use of wine or brandy in infantile typhoid and typhus, see Hillier on *Diseases of Children*, a most admirable work.

upon himself, is rightly considered deficient
in recuperative vigour. When such occasions
come, most persons instinctively seek aid from
alcohol ; and it helps them because it is an
imparter, or at least an economizer, of nervous
force. The fact that it is resorted to, when
supreme exertion is demanded, shows that it
is recognized as a strength-saver, if not as a
strength-giver. Our inquiry into its food-
action will show that it is both the one and
the other.

Thus far we have considered alcohol only
as an agent which affects the nutrition of the
nerves. Whether it be also a food or not
does not essentially alter the question of its
evil or beneficent influence upon the system.
As we saw in our chapter on Tobacco, the
human organism needs, for its proper nutrition, stimulus as well as food,—force as well
as material. No conclusion in physiology is
better established than that narcotic-stimulants increase the supply of force while they

diminish the waste of material;[19] and it is by virtue of this peculiarity that they will often sustain the organism in the absence of food. Tobacco is not food, but if you give a starving man a pipe to smoke it will take him much longer to die. Opium and coca are not foods ; but they will sometimes support life when no true aliment can be procured. The action of alcohol is similar to that of these substances, but immeasurably more effective. None of the inferior narcotic-stimulants is at all comparable with alcohol in the degree of its food-replacing power. We read that tobacco and coca will enable a man to go several days without anything to eat; and we interpret this result as due to the waste-retarding action of these substances. But when we find that alcohol will support life for weeks and months, we

---

[19] See Chambers, *Digestion and its Derangements,* p. 249 ; and in general, Johnston, Von Bibra, and the paper of Dr. Hammond above referred to.

can no longer be content with such an explanation. When we recollect that Cornaro
lived healthily for fifty-eight years upon
twelve ounces of light food and fourteen
ounces of wine *per diem*,[20] and reflect upon
the large proportion of alcoholic drink in
this diet, the suspicion is forced upon us
that alcohol is not only a true stimulant but
also a true food.

Mr. Parton of course asserts that alcoholic
drinks do not nourish the body, and denies
to them the title of foods. He begins by
quoting Liebig's assertion " that as much
flour or meal as can lie on the point of a
table-knife is more nutritious than nine quarts
of the best Bavarian beer." Whereupon the
reader, who is perhaps not familiar with the
history of physiological controversy, thinks
at once that Liebig's great authority is op-
posed to the opinion that alcohol is food.
Nothing could be further from the truth.

[20] Carpenter, *Human Physiology*, p. 887.

Perhaps nothing in Mr. Parton's book shows more forcibly the danger of "cramming" a subject instead of studying it. When Liebig wrote the above sentence, he believed that foods might be sharply divided into two classes,—those which nourish, and those which keep up the heat of the body. He believed that no foods except those which contain nitrogen can nourish the tissues; and he therefore excluded not only alcohol, *but fat, starch and sugar also*, from the class of nutritious substances. But Liebig was far from believing that alcohol is not food. On the contrary he distinctly classed it with fat, starch and sugar, as a *heat-producing food,*— a fact which Mr. Parton, if he knows it, takes good care not to quote! But this twofold classification of foods has for several years been known to be unsound. It has been shown that all true foods are more or less nutritious, and that all are more or less heat-producing. Starch and sugar have maintained their places in the class of nutritive materials from which Liebig tried to exclude them, and we have now to see whether the same can be said of the closely kindred substance, alcohol.

Mr. Parton thinks he has proved that alcohol cannot be food, when he has asserted that it is not chemically transformed within the body. As soon as it is taken, he tells us, lungs, skin and kidneys all set busily to work to expel it, and they send it out just as it came in: *therefore* it is an enemy. Now all this may be said of water. Water is not chemically changed within the body; as soon as we drink it, lungs, skin and kidneys begin busily to expel it; and it goes out just as good water as it came in. Nevertheless, water is one of the most essential elements of nutrition.

But it is by no means certain that alcohol is not transformed within the body. It is neither certain nor probable. Mr. Parton

relies upon the experiments of Messrs. Lallemand, Duroy, and Perrin, who in 1860
thought they had demonstrated that *all* the
alcohol taken into the system comes out
again, *as* alcohol, through the lungs, skin
and kidneys. By applying the very delicate
chromic acid test, these gentlemen appeared
to prove that appreciable quantities of alcohol always begin to be excreted very soon
after the dose has been received by the
stomach, and continue to pass off for many
hours. "They failed, after repeated attempts,
to discover the intermediate compounds into
which alcohol had been represented as trans-
forming itself before its final change; and, on
the other hand, they detected *unchanged* alcohol everywhere in the body hours after it had
been taken; they found the substance in the
blood, and in all the tissues, but especially
in the brain and the nervous centres generally, and in the liver."[21]   Mr. Parton has, it

[21] Anstie, op. cit., p. 359.

would appear, read their book, and he is fully persuaded by it that "if you take into your system an ounce of alcohol, the whole ounce leaves the system within forty-eight hours, just as good alcohol as it went in." These experiments, moreover, "produced the remarkable effect of causing the editor of a leading periodical to confess to the public that he was not infallible." The *Westminster Review*, it seems, in 1861, retracted the opinions which it had expressed in 1855, "concerning the *rôle* of alcohol in the animal body." The *Westminster Review* has now an opportunity to retract its recantations; for in 1863, these experiments were subjected to a searching criticism by M. Baudot, which resulted in thoroughly invalidating the conclusions supposed to flow from them.[22] The case is an interesting one, as showing afresh

---

[22] Baudot, *De la Destruction de l'Alcool dans l'Organisme, Union Médicale,* Nov. et Déc., 1863. See also the elaborate criticism in Anstie, op. cit., pp. 358—370.

the utter impossibility of getting at the truth concerning alcohol, without paying attention to the difference in the behaviour of large and small quantities.

The researches of Bouchardat and Sandras,[23] and of Duchek,[24] have rendered it probable that, if alcohol undergoes any digestive transformation, it is first changed into aldehyde, from which are successively formed acetic acid, oxalic acid and water, and carbonic acid.[25] But this transformation, like any other digestive process, cannot go on unless the nervous system is in good working order. Now when a narcotic dose of alcohol is taken, the flow of gastric juice is prevented by local paralysis of the nerve-fibres distributed to the stomach. What then must hap-

---

[23] *De la Digestion des Boissons Alcooliques*, in *Annales de Chimie et de Physique*, 1847, tom. xxi.

[24] *Ueber das Verhalten des Alkohols im thierischen Organismus*, in *Vierteljahrsschrift für die praktische Heilkunde*, Prague, 1833.

[25] See Moleschott, *Circulation de la Vie*, tom. ii. p. 6.

pen? Solid food may remain undigested, in
the stomach;[26] but liquid alcohol is easily
absorbable, and has two ways of exit,—one
through the portal system into the liver, the
other through the lacteals into the general
circulation, by which it will be carried chiefly
to the organ which receives most blood,—
namely, the brain. *It is thus probable that no
alcohol can be transformed after narcosis begins.*
But the absorbed alcohol, loading the circulation, begins at once to be excreted. Paralysis of the renal plexus of the sympathetic
sets up a rapid diuresis, and considerable
amounts of the volatile liquid escape through
the lungs and skin. In examining, therefore,
a drunken man or dog, we need not, on any

---

[26] So decisive is the paralyzing power of a narcotic
dose of alcohol upon the stomach in some cases, that
we have seen a drunken man vomit scarcely altered
food which, it appeared, had been eaten fourteen hours
before. The sum and substance of the above argument is that, as the narcotic dose of alcohol prevents
the digestion of other food, it will also prevent the
digestion of itself.

theory, expect to find the intermediate products of alcoholic transformation; we must expect to find large quantities of undigested alcohol in the circulation, and notably in the brain and liver; and we need not be surprised if we detect unchanged alcohol in the excretions. *Our experiment will not show that alcohol cannot be assimilated; it will only show how serious is the damage inflicted by a narcotic dose, in checking assimilation.* Now all this applies with force to the experiments of Messrs. Lallemand, Duroy and Perrin. In their experiments, these gentlemen always tried intoxicating doses; thus paralyzing at the outset the whole digestive tract, *and preventing the formation of those transformed products which they afterward vainly tried to discover.* As so often happens in experimenting upon the enormously complex human organism, they began by creating abnormal conditions which rendered their conclusions inapplicable to the healthy body

A further criticism by M. Baudot, supported by renewed experiments, is still more
decisive. M. Baudot justly observes that in
order to substantiate their conclusions, Messrs.
Lallemand, Duroy and Perrin should have at
least been able, with their excessively delicate
tests, to discover in the excretions *a large part*
of the alcohol which had been taken into the
system. This, however, they never did. In
all cases, the amount of alcohol recovered was
very small, and bore but a trifling proportion
to the amount which had been taken. According to these physiologists, the elimination
always takes place chiefly through the kidneys.
But M. Baudot, in a series of elaborate experiments, has proved that, unless the dose has
been excessive, *no sensible amount of alcohol re-
appears in the kidney-excretions for more than
twenty-four hours.* The quantity is so minute
that the alcoometer is not in the least affected
by it, and it requires the chromic acid test

even to reveal its presence. Similar results
have been obtained by experiments upon the
breath.

Finally, the gravest doubts have been
thrown upon the trustworthiness of the chromic acid test relied on by Messrs. Lallemand,
Duroy and Perrin. It is considered possible,
by good chemical authority, that the reactions
in the test-apparatus, which they attributed to
the escaping alcohol, may equally well have
been caused by some of the results of alcoholic transformation. For reasons above given,
however, it is probable that in cases of narcosis some alcohol always escapes. When we
reflect upon its absorbability and its ready
solubility in water, it seems likely beforehand
that a considerable quantity must escape. But
all that these able Frenchmen can be said to
have accomplished, is the demonstration of the
fact·that when you take into your system a
greater quantity of alcohol than the system

can manage, a part of it is expelled in the same state in which it entered. And this may be said of other kinds of food.

These experiments have, therefore, instead of settling the question, left it substantially just where it was before. But we have now a more remarkable set of facts to contemplate. In many cases of typhoid fever, acute bronchitis, pneumonia, erysipelas, and diphtheria, occurring in Dr. Anstie's practice, it was found that the stomach could be made to retain nothing but wine or brandy. Upon these alcoholic drinks, therefore, the patients were entirely sustained for periods sometimes reaching a month in duration.[27] In nearly every case convalescence was rapid, and the emaciation was much slighter than usual: the quality of the flesh was also observed to be remarkably

[27] In typhoid and typhus the "poison-line" of alcohol is shifted, so that large quantities may be taken without risk of narcosis. Women, in this condition, have been known to consume 36 oz. of brandy (containing 18 oz. of alcohol) *per diem.*

good. Dr. Slack, of Liverpool, had two female patients who, loathing ordinary food, maintained life and tolerable vigour for more than three months upon alcoholic drinks alone. Mr. Nisbet reports "the case of a child affected with marasmus, who subsisted for three months on sweet whisky and water alone, and then recovered; and that of another child, who lived entirely upon Scotch ale for a fortnight, and then recovered his appetite for common things." Many similar examples might be cited.

It may be said that alcohol maintained these persons by retarding the waste of the tissues. This is no doubt an admissible supposition. There is no doubt that alcohol, by its waste-retarding action, will postpone for some time the day of death from starvation.[23] But to this action there must be some limit.

---

[23] It is not certain, however, that alcoholic drinks, as usually taken, materially retard the waste of tissue. These drinks contain but from 2 to 50 per cent of alcohol; the remainder being chiefly water, which is a great accelerator of waste. The weight-sustaining power of brandy, or

Though the waste is retarded, it is not wholly
stopped.   Though there is relatively less waste,
there is still absolutely large waste.   The mere
act of keeping up respiration necessitates a
considerable destruction of tissue.   Then the
temperature of the body must be kept very
near 98° Fahrenheit, or life will suddenly
cease; and the maintenance of this heat involves a great consumption of tissue.   Now
this waste, under the most favourable circumstances, will soon destroy life, unless it is
balanced by actual repair.   You may diminish the draught on your furnace as much as
you please,—the fire will shortly go out unless
fresh coal is added.   Upon these points the
data are more or less precise.   The amount
of waste material daily excreted from the body,
under ordinary circumstances, is a little more
than seven pounds.[29]   Of this the greater part

especially of wine and ale, can, therefore, perhaps be hardly
accounted for without admitting a true food-action.

[29] Dalton, *Human Physiology*, p. 363.

is water, the quantity of carbon being about twelve ounces, and the quantity of nitrogenous matter about five ounces.[30] To make up for this waste we usually require at least two and a half pounds of solid, and three pints of liquid, food.[31] In Dr. Hammond's experiments, the weight-sustaining power of the alcohol taken seems to have amounted to four or five ounces.[32] It will be seen, therefore, that in spite of any stimulant effect of alcohol upon nutrition, unless at least ten or twelve ounces of nitrogenous or carbonaceous matter be eaten daily, the weight of the body must rapidly diminish.

Now the experiments of Chossat have demonstrated that no animal can suddenly lose more than two-fifths of its normal weight without dying of starvation. If a man, therefore,

---

[30] Payen, *Substances Alimentaires*, p. 482.

[31] The liquid food may be taken in the shape of free water, or of water contained in the tissues of succulent vegetables. See Pereira, *Treatise on Food and Diet*, p. 277.

[32] *Physiological Memoirs*, Philadelphia, 1863, p. 48.

7

weigh 150 lbs., for him 90 lbs. is the starvation-point; as soon as he reaches that weight he dies. Usually, indeed, death occurs before this degree of emaciation can have been attained,—in most cases, on the fifth or sixth day; though there are a few authentic instances of persons who have lived for twelve, and even sixteen, days before finally succumbing.

In view of these facts, we are willing to grant that people may in rare cases live for three months on their own tissues, if waste be duly retarded. We are willing to grant it, though we do not believe it. But we are not prepared to admit that this process can go on for six months or a year; and we believe that the cases now to be cited can in nowise be got rid of by such an interpretation.

Mr. Nisbet mentions the case of a man who lived for seven months entirely on spirit and water. At Wavertree, a young man afflicted with heart-disease lived for five years principally, and for two years solely, on brandy. His allowance was at first six ounces, afterward a pint, *per diem.* His weight was not materially decreased, when, at the end of the five years, he died of his disease. But the next case is still more remarkable. Dr. Inman had a lady-patient, about twenty-five years old, plump, active and florid, but somewhat deficient in power of endurance. "This lady had two large and healthy children in succession, whom she successfully nursed. On each occasion she became much exhausted, the appetite wholly failed, and she was compelled to live solely on bitter ale and brandy and water; on this regimen she kept up her good looks, her activity and her nursing, and went on this way for about twelve months; the nervous system was by this time thoroughly exhausted, *yet there was no emaciation,* nor was there entire prostration of muscular power."[33]

---

[33] Anstie, op. cit. p. 388.

For the accuracy of this statement there
is to be had the testimony of Dr. Inman, the
attendant physician, as well as that " of the
lady's husband, of mutual friends occasionally
residing in the house with her, of her mother,
of her sisters, and of her nurse." We have
apparently no alternative but to believe it;
and if it is true, it is certainly decisive. It
is nothing less than an *experimentum crucis.*
The suggestion that this lady might have
kept up her normal activity while nursing
children, for a whole year, with no aliment
except her own tissues and the water and
vegetable matter contained in her ale and
brandy, is too absurd to need refutation. The
thing is an utter impossibility. Moreover,
not being emaciated at the end of the year,
she had probably been consuming her own
tissues but very little. Her weight, her muscular activity, and the natural heat of her
body, could have been sustained by nothing
but the alcohol; which thus appears as a

true food, at once nourishing, strength-giving, and heat-producing.

This conclusion is further re-enforced by the numerous cases on record of persons who have lived actively for many years upon a diet of alcoholic liquor accompanied by a quantity of solid food notoriously inadequate to support life. The case of Cornaro is outdone by some of those quoted by Dr. Anstie, as having occurred under his own observation. Of twelve cases which are described in detail, the most remarkable is that of a man aged 83, whose diet for twenty years had consisted of one bottle of gin and one small fragment of toasted bread daily. This old fellow, says Dr. Anstie, "would have been of little service as a practical illustration of the bodily harm wrought by drinking, being in truth rather an unusually active and vigorous person for his time of life." Probably the old man was not narcotized by his daily bottle of gin; or he would, long before the twenty years had

elapsed, have shown symptoms of nervous disease. In most of these cases of abnormal
diet, there occurs after a while a general
breaking down of the nerve-centres, shown in
delirium tremens, epileptic fits, or a sudden
stroke of paralysis. They are not quoted,
therefore, as examples to be followed, but as
very important items of evidence in favour
of the opinion that alcohol is food.

Taking all these considerations together,
we believe it to be tolerably well made out
that alcohol, whether changed within the body
or not, is a true food, which nourishes, warms
and strengthens. And Dr. Brinton, in the
following passage, declares it to be, in many
cases, a necessary food. " That teetotalism
is compatible with health, it needs no elaborate facts to establish; but if we take the
customary life of those constituting the masses
of our inhabitants of towns, we shall find
reason to wait before we assume that this
result will extend to our population at large.

And, in respect to experience, it is singular how few healthy teetotalers are to be met with in our ordinary inhabitants of cities. Glancing back over the many years during which this question has been forced upon the author by his professional duties, he may estimate that he has sedulously examined not less than 50,000 to 70,000 persons, including many thousands in perfect health. Wishing, and even expecting to find it otherwise, he is obliged to confess that he has hitherto met with but very few perfectly healthy middle-aged persons, successfully pursuing any arduous metropolitan calling under teetotal habits. On the other hand, he has known many total abstainers, whose apparently sound constitutions have given way with unusual and frightful rapidity when attacked by a casual sickness." "This," says an English reviewer of the French experiments, "is quite in accordance with what I have myself observed, and with what I can gather from other medical men ; and it speaks

volumes concerning the way in which we
ought to regard alcohol. If, indeed, it be a
fact that in a certain high state of civilization
men require to take alcohol every day, in
some shape or other, under penalty of breaking down prematurely in their work, it is idle
to appeal to a set of imperfect chemical or
physiological experiments, and to decide, on
their evidence, that we ought to call alcohol
a medicine or a poison, but not a food. I am
obliged to declare that the chemical evidence
is as yet insufficient to give any complete explanation of its exact manner of action upon
the system; but that the practical facts are as
striking as they could well be, and that there
can be no mistake about them. And I have
thought it proper that, while highly-coloured
statements of the results of the new French
researches are being somewhat disingenuously
placed before the lay public, there should not
be a total silence on the part of those members of the profession who do not see them-

selves called upon to yield to the mere force of agitation."[34] If this view of the case, which so strongly recommends itself to the mind of the practical physician, be the true one, we are forced to regard teetotalism, considered not in its moral but in its physiological aspects, as a dietetic heresy nearly akin to vegetarianism. Man can do without wine, as he can do without meat; but the rational course is to adopt that diet from which we can obtain the greatest amount of available vital power.

But even if we were to give up the doctrine that alcohol is a true food, the great indisputed and indisputable fact of its stimulant value would still remain. Tobacco neither nourishes the body nor warms it; yet it enables us to earn our daily bread with less fatigue, and to support the inces-

---

[34] Brinton, *Treatise on Food and Digestion;* and *Cornhill Magazine*, Sept. 1862; cited in the pamphlet of Gov. Andrew, above-mentioned.

sant trials of life with a more even spirit.
The value of alcohol as a stimulant is inferior only to that of tobacco; or perhaps,
for general purposes, it is quite unsurpassed.
It compensates for the occasionally inevitable incapacity of ordinary food to maintain
due nutrition; and in this way enables us
to work longer, and with a lighter heart, and
with less fear of ultimate depression.   It
bridges over the pitfalls which the complicated exigencies of modern life are constantly digging for us.   Warm-hearted but weak-
headed radicalism may imagine a utopian
state of things in which money will grow on
bushes and every one mind the moral law,
and digestion be always easy, and vexation
infrequent, and " artificial" stimulus unneces-
sary; but this is not the state of things amid
which we live.   A modern man cannot, if he
does his duty, secure to himself the enjoyment of such a state.   There are times when
he must sacrifice a little of his own round per-

fection, if it be only to lend a· helping hand
to his neighbour. A kind of valetudinarian
philosophy is now afloat, which says, Look out,
above all things, for your own physical wel-
fare. This philosophy contains a truth, but
as usually manifested it is nothing but the
result of a morbid self-consciousness. Duty
sometimes requires that we should cease cod-
dling ourselves, and go to work, unless we
would see some cause suffer which interests
other men, living and to come, besides ourselves. We must sometimes run to put the
fire out, even if we do thereby lose our dinner,
and interfere with the stomach's requirements.
It is useless, then, to talk about agents which
"support us in doing wrong," when, from the
very constitution of the world and of society,
we can no more go exactly "right" than we
can draw a line which shall be mathemati-
cally straight. It is useless to speculate about
an ideal society in which men can dispense
with the agents which economize their ner-

vous strength, when we find as a historical fact that no nation has ever existed which has been able to dispense with those agents. As long as there are inequalities in the daily ratio of waste and repair to be rectified, so long we shall get along better with wine than without it. For this, looked at from the widest possible point of view, is the legitimate function of alcohol,—*to diminish the necessary friction of living.*

This too is the view of Liebig: "As a restorative, a means of refreshment when the powers of life are exhausted, of giving animation and energy where man has to struggle with days of sorrow, as a means of correction and compensation where misproportion occurs in nutrition, wine is surpassed by no product of nature or of art. . . . In no part of Germany do the apothecaries' establishments bring so low a price as in the rich cities on the Rhine; for there wine is the universal medicine of the healthy as well as the sick. It is considered as milk for the aged." [35]

This is also the view of Dr. Anstie. Comparing the action of alcohol upon the organism with that of chloroform and sulphuric ether, he observes : "It seems as if the former were intended to be the medicine of those ailments which are engendered of the *necessary* every-day evils of civilized life, and has therefore been made attractive to the senses, and easily retained in the tissues, and in various ways approving itself to our judgment as *a food ;* while the others, which are more rarely needed for their stimulant properties, and are chiefly valuable for their beneficent temporary poisonous action, by the help of which painful operations are sustained with impunity, are in great measure deprived of these attractions, and of their facilities for entering and remaining in the system." [26] Apart from its implied teleology,

---

[35] Liebig, *Letters on Chemistry*, p. 454.
[36] Anstie, op. cit. p. 401.

this passage contains the gist of the whole matter.

As for the Coming Man, whom Mr. Parton appears to regard as a sort of pugilist or Olympic athlete, we suppose he will undoubtedly. have to exercise his brain sometimes, he will have to study, think and plan, he will have responsibilities to shoulder, his digestion will not always be preserved at its maximum of efficiency, his powers of endurance will sometimes be tried to the utmost. The period in the future when "we shall have changed all this" is altogether too remote to affect our present conclusion; which is that the Coming Man, so long as he is a member of a complex, civilized society, will continue to use, with profit as well as pleasure, the two universal stimulants, Alcohol and Tobacco.

APPENDIX.

Bibliography of Tobacco.

For the benefit of those readers who may feel interested in this subject, the following list is added, of the principal works which have been written on the effects of tobacco. The older ones have, of course, little scientific value, yet they are often interesting and suggestive. They usually made the best use of the science of their time, which is more than can be said of some of the later treatises.

Baumann: Dissertatio de Tabaci virtutibus. Basil, 1579.
Everart: De herba Panacea. Antwerp, 1583.
Ziegler: Taback von dem gar heilsamen Wundkraute Nicotiana. Zurich, 1616.
Marradon: Dialogo del uso del Tabaco. Seville, 1618.
De Castro: Historia de las virtudes y propriedades de Tabacco. Cordova, 1620.
Thorius: Hymnus Tabaci. Leyden, 1622.
Neander: Tabacologia. Leyden, 1622.
Scriverius: Saturnalia, seu de usu et abusu Tabaci. Haarlem, 1628.
Braun: Quæstio medica de fumo Tabaci. Marburg, 1628.
Aguilar: Contra il mal uso del Tabaco. Cordova, 1633.

Frankenius : Dissertatio de virtutibus Nicotianæ. Upsal, 1633.

Ostendorf : Traité de l'usage et de l'abus du Tabac. Paris, 1636.

Venner : Via recta ad vitam longam. London, 1637. (See p. 363, for an entertaining discourse on Tobacco.)

Ferrant : Traité du Tabac en sternutatoire. Bourges, 1645.

Cuffari : I biasimi del Tabacco. Palermo, 1645.

Vitaliani : De abusu Tabaci. Rome, 1650.

Tapp : Oratio de Tabaco. Helmstadt, 1653.

Balde : Satyra contra abusum Tabaci. Munich, 1657.

Magnenus : Exercitationes XIV. de Tabaco. Ticino, 1658.

Rumsey : Organum Salutis. London, 1659.

Paulli : Commentarius de abusu Tabaci Americanorum veteri. Argentorat. 1665.

Baillard : Discours du Tabac. Paris, 1668.

De Prade : Histoire du Tabac. Paris, 1677.

Van Bontekoe : Korte verhandeling van t' menschenleven gezondheit, ziekte en dood, etc. s' Gravenhagen, 1684.

Worp Beintema : Tabacologia, ofte korte verhandelinge over de Toback. s' Gravenhagen, 1690.

Fagon : Dissertatio an ex Tabaci usu frequenti vita brevior. Paris, 1699.

Brunet : Le bon usage du Tabac en poudre. Paris, 1700.

Della Fabra : Dissertatio de animi affectibus, etc. Ferrara, 1702.

Manara : De moderando Tabaci usu in Europæis. Madrid, 1702.

Nicolicchia : Uso ed abuso del Tabacco. Palermo, 1710.

Keyl: Dissertatio num Nicotianæ herbæ usu levis notæ maculam contrahat. Leipsic, 1715.

Cohausen: Pica nasi, seu de Tabaci sternutatorii abusu et noxa. Amsterdam, 1716.

Meier: Tabacomania. Nordhaus, 1720.

——: A Dissertation on the Use and Abuse of Tobacco in Relation to Smoaking, Chewing, and taking of Snuff. London, 1720.

Plaz: De Tabaco sternutatorio. Leipsic, 1727.

Stahl: Dissertatio de Tabaci effectibus salutaribus et nocivis. Erfurt, 1732.

Maloet: Dissertatio an a Tabaco, naribus assumpto, peculiaris quædam cephalalgiæ species, aliique effectus. Paris, 1733.

Alberti: De Tabaci fumum sugente theologo. Halle, 1743.

Garbenfeld: Dissertatio de Tabaci usu et abusu. Argent. 1744.

Beck: De suctione fumi Tabaci. Altdorf, 1745.

Büchner: De genuinis viribus Tabaci. Halle, 1746.

Herment: Dissertatio an post cibum fumus Tabaci, etc. Paris, 1749.

De la Sone: Dissertatio an Tabacum homini sit lentum venenum. Paris, 1751.

Ferrein: Dissertatio an ex Tabaci usu frequenti vitæ summa brevior. Paris, 1753.

Petitmaitre: De usu et abusu Nicotianæ. Basil, 1756.

Triller: Disputatio de Tabaci ptarmici abusu, affectus ventriculi causa. Wittenberg, 1761.

Cuntira: De viribus medicis Nicotianæ ejusque usu et abusu. Vienna, 1777.

Hamilton: De Nicotianæ viribus in Medicina et de ejus malis effectibus in usu communi et domestico. Edinburgh, 1779.

Clarke: A dissertation on the Use and Abuse of Tobacco. London, 1797.

Szerlecki: Monographie über den Tabak. Stuttgart, 1840.

Stahmann: Cigarre, Pfeife, und Dose. Quedlinburg, 1852.

Baldwin: Evils of Tobacco. New York, 1854.

Trall: Tobacco, its History, etc. New York, 1854.

——: Discours contre l'usage du Tabac. Nantes, 1854.

——: Discours en faveur du Tabac. Nantes, 1854.

Tiedemann: Geschichte des Tabaks. Frankfort. 1854.

Vlaanderen: Over den Tabak, bijzonder over zijne on bewerktuigde bestanddeelen. Utrecht, 1854.

Felip: El Tabaco. Madrid, 1854.

Hortmann: Der Tabaksbau. Emmerich, 1855.

Von Bibra: Die Narkotischen Genussmittel und der Mensch. Nürnberg, 1855.

Tognola: Riflessioni intorno all' uso igenico del Tabacco. Padua, 1855.

——: A Commentary on the Influence which the Use of Tobacco exerts on the Human Constitution. Sydney, 1856.

Jarnatowsky: De Nicotiana ejusque abusu. Berlin, 1856.

Asencio: Reflexiones sobre la renta del Tabaco. Madrid, 1856.

Hammond: The Physiological Action of Alcohol and Tobacco upon the Human Organism. American Journal of Medical Sciences. October, 1856.

Budgett: The Tobacco Question, Morally, Socially, and Physically. London, 1857.

Cavendish: A few Words in Defence of Tobacco. London, 1857.

Jeumont: Du Tabac, de son Usage, de ses Effets, etc. Paris, 1857.

Lizars: On the Use and Abuse of Tobacco. London, 1857.

Steinmetz: Tobacco. London, 1857.

Alexandre: Contre l'abus du Tabac. Amiens, 1857.

Fermond: Monographie du Tabac. Paris, 1857.

Koller: Der Tabac. Augsburg, 1858.

Prescott: Tobacco and its Adulterations. London, 1858.

Schmid: Der Tabak als wichtige Culturpflanze. Weimar, 1858.

Demoor: Du Tabac. Brussels, 1858.

Mourgues: Traité de la Culture du Tabac. Paris, 1859.

Morand: Essai sur l'Hygiène du Tabac. Epinal, 1859.

Fairholt: Tobacco, its History and Associations. London, 1859.

Cheever: On Tobacco. Atlantic Monthly, August, 1860.